LECTURE NOTES ON
PAEDIATRICS

LECTURE NOTES ON
PAEDIATRICS

S. R. MEADOW

MA, BM, FRCP, DCH, DRCOG
Senior Lecturer in
Paediatrics and Child Health,
University of Leeds; Honorary
Consultant Paediatrician,
Leeds Area Health
Authority (Teaching)

R. W. SMITHELLS

MB, FRCP, FRCP(E), DCH
Professor of Paediatrics and
Child Health, University of Leeds;
Honorary Consultant Paediatrician,
Leeds Area Health
Authority (Teaching)

SECOND EDITION

Blackwell Scientific Publications

OXFORD LONDON EDINBURGH
MELBOURNE

© 1973, 1975 Blackwell Scientific Publications
Osney Mead, Oxford,
85 Marylebone High Street, London W1M 3DE,
9 Forrest Road, Edinburgh,
P.O. Box 9, North Balwyn, Victoria, Australia.

ISBN 0 632 00397 9

First published 1973
Revised second printing 1974
Second edition 1975

Distributed in the United States of America by
J. B. Lippincott Company, Philadelphia,
and in Canada by
J. B. Lippincott Company of Canada Ltd, Toronto

Printed in Great Britain at the Alden Press, Oxford

CONTENTS

PREFACE TO THE SECOND EDITION

The task of producing a second edition has been enjoyable because it has confirmed our belief that paediatrics is one of the most dynamic areas of contemporary medicine. In the brief interval since our first edition there have been important advances. The advances begin with those of the perinatal period—amniocentesis and prenatal detection of abnormalities are now routine; extend into infancy with the resurgence of interest and new research findings concerning infant feeding; and lead on to the more precise techniques now available for the management of ill children, and the reconstructed services for families in our society.

We have made broader alteration than was possible in the revised first edition, and have been able to incorporate most of the helpful suggestions from our colleagues and students.

Many of the chapters have been extensively rewritten. Though the general aspects of history taking and examination remain in the first chapter, details of the examination of each system are given in the chapter dealing with that system. Therapeutics has been expanded into a new chapter of its own. Some earlier omissions, for instance sleep disorders, are put right. However, we have tried to prevent the book expanding by pruning as well as planting.

A short bibliography has been added at the end of each chapter. It includes some of the books, articles and chapters which we found particularly helpful, but we hope it will not drive any students still further away from the wards and clinics, for we remain convinced that the best way to learn paediatrics is to talk and play with children, examine them and listen to their parents.

Roy Meadow
Dick Smithells

Leeds, 1975

PREFACE TO THE FIRST EDITION

Paediatrics concerns the health and illness of children. Children make up more than one-fifth of our population and an even higher proportion of a general practitioner's working day. It is often in childhood that the patterns of adult health and disease have their origins. Paediatrics rubs shoulders with education and with the social services. It is concerned with children and their families first, and with disease second.

Medical education is a continuing process which starts at school and should not end before retirement. The pre-registration year ensures that the new medical student is not 'let loose upon the public'. Today's medical students should therefore be expected to absorb less factual material than did their ancestors. This is a small book, intended to live in the pocket of a white coat rather than on a bookshelf. It describes the pattern of childhood growth and development and conditions which are either common, important or interesting. This factual framework is set against the changing pattern of paediatric practice, the services available for children and the needs of society.

Our aim has been to provide a framework of paediatric knowledge sufficient for the medical student during the paediatric appointment; but it must be grafted on to preliminary experience of adult medicine and surgery. We have deliberately placed more emphasis on diagnosis than on treatment; therapeutic details are best learned by caring for sick children.

For medical students who use this book, far more important than further reading is the need to spend time and trouble getting to know children, and developing the techniques of examining children and talking to them and their parents. This applies also to the many other groups who work with children—therapists, nurses and health visitors—for whom we hope this book will provide a useful supplement to their lectures and their work.

ACKNOWLEDGMENTS

We thank our colleagues for their advice and help, and Miss Angela Tempest for her efficient and intelligent secretarial work in preparing the manuscript.

The figures were drawn by Mr H.Grayshon Lumby, MSIA, and most of the photographs were prepared by the Department of Medical Photography at the University of Leeds and United Leeds Hospitals.

We are grateful to a number of colleagues who have helped with the illustrations, particularly Mrs G.Levell, Dr J.M. Littlewood and Professor V.Dubowitz. The following authors and publishers kindly allowed us to reproduce illustrations:

Figure 9. J.M.Tanner, Institute of Child Health, Guilford Street, London W.C.1.

Figure 61: F.T.W.Miller, *Growing up in Newcastle Upon Tyne*, 1960, Oxford University Press, London.

Appendix 4: R.M.Blizzard, *Diagnosis and Treatment of Endocrine Disorders in Childhood*, 3rd edition, 1965, Charles C.Thomas, Springfield, Illinois.

The second edition owes much to our most capable and thoughtful assistant Miss Angela Fergusson, to whom we are grateful.

Chapter 1

THE CHILD AS A PATIENT

HISTORY TAKING

The child's history covers the same ground as that of an adult patient, with some important additions. The start is similar. We need to know the **name, age and sex** of the patient and their reason for consulting us. Find out and write on the notes what the child is called at home, e.g. 'Larry'. This avoids anyone greeting him with an unfamiliar formal name—'Good Morning Lawrence'.

The **history of the present condition** (including a review of the systems) will usually be obtained from the parent, though any child who can talk may be able to contribute additional useful information. A five-year-old may agree to 'put your hand where it hurts'. Older children should be seen on their own for a few minutes with the parent out of the room. This allows direct doctor–child communication, increases the child's self-confidence and ensures better co-operation with future management. It also enables the doctor to speak to the parent alone without the child feeling slighted: 'Please will you wait outside while I talk with your mummy, and then she'll wait outside while I talk with you.'

School is the equivalent of an adult's employment. School attendance and progress are important parameters, and the name of the school should be noted so that a report from the school teacher can be obtained if necessary.

That ubiquitous student catch phrase 'No diabetes, epilepsy or TB' appearing under **family history** is usually irrelevant; what must be recorded are: (1) The number and ages of the siblings and parents, (2) Whether any other member of the family has or has had the same condition as the child—whether it be a rash and fever (? has the child caught the same infection), or seven fingers on each hand (? has the child an inherited condition which runs in the family), (3) What diseases the parents and close relatives have had, in order to allay needless worries. The parents may worry that their child's stomach ache is caused by stomach cancer, because grandma recently died with it, (4) The presence or absence of consanguinity should be recorded, because rare inherited conditions are more likely if the parents are related by common ancestry.

The **perinatal history** should provide details of the pregnancy (its length, any abnormalities, any maternal illnesses), delivery and first few days of life (the birth weight, asphyxia, any need of incubation or special care). A variety of conditions including cerebral palsy and mental subnormality may originate from problems occurring before, during or soon after birth.

Details of **previous diseases** should also include details of previous immunizations: first, since it may help to exclude a suspected condition, and secondly to identify those families in need of advice about further immunization.

The **developmental history** is almost unique to paediatrics. It is an important part of the history particularly for young children or handicapped children. It includes details of the milestones, the times at which skills such as walking and talking were acquired by the child (Chapter 5).

To obtain a good **social history** one must establish rapport with the parents and talk with them about their life, their home, their work and their problems. Three particular areas must be explored which have a direct influence on the child's development: (1) The family composition: are the mother and father living together, or is this a single parent family who in our society are 'the poorest of the poor'. (2) The financial situation: is the family economically viable with a regular income, or are they dependent on grants from the Social Services Department. (3) Housing: have they a home of their own, and if so what sort; or are they living with relatives or in a hostel? Satisfactory housing should have not more than 1.5 persons per room, and a supply of hot water.

EXAMINATION

The rigid rules that have been learnt for examining adults have to be bent when applied to small babies, frightened toddlers and nervous children. The young child has to be charmed and seduced before he will allow a useful examination. A baby responds to comforting noises and smiles, an older child to gentle friendly talk and play.

Examination of the school child is not difficult. Most are cooperative and confident provided a parent is there. Those over the age of 10 may prefer more privacy, but although they may prefer to be examined without their parent watching they are usually comforted by their nearby presence.

Pre-school children are more difficult. The doctor must be an opportunist, adapting his examination to the openings that present. The infant should be examined as he allows you to; if he is quiet listen to the heart, if his eyes are open look at his eyes. It is useless demanding at the start 'remove all the clothes' if this is going to result in prolonged crying—small children don't like taking their clothes off; it's cold, their vests are tight and hurt their ears as they're pulled off, they feel insecure. More information is obtained from a partly clothed contented child than from a screaming naked one, so it is best to leave removal of clothes to the end of the examination.

Children worry about any instruments so these need to be explained and a running commentary kept up for the benefit of child and parent. The grim-faced silent doctor spells doom, whilst the calm friendly one radiates optimistic confidence with his 'Your hair is nice', 'Your heart is strong', 'Your blood pressure is very healthy'. Gaiety may be out of place when a child is ill but it is better to be buoyant and cheerful than unresponsive and dull.

The techniques for examining the different systems are given in the chapters about those systems. All new patients should have their height and weight measured and checked against the normal range for their age. Poor growth or low weight relative to height may be a sign of serious illness. Note is taken of the child's cleanliness and clothes, and of evidence of scalp infestation or bitten nails that may be signs of other problems. Routine urine examination (page 183) is also obligatory. The temperature is

3

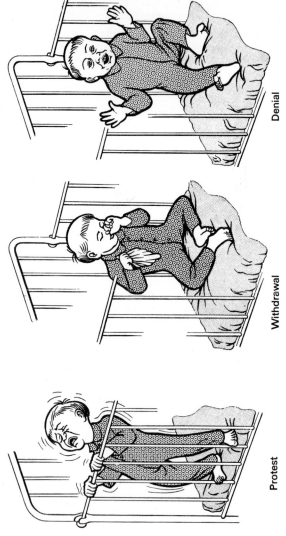

Protest　　　　**Withdrawal**　　　　**Denial**

Fig. 1. A young child's response to separation from his mother. He eventually denies the presence of his mother and superficially appears happy.

usually taken rectally during the first year of life, in the axilla up to the age of 5, and orally in school children.

CHILDREN IN HOSPITAL

The hazards of illness are obvious to everyone; the hazards of hospitalization and of parent/child separation are less obvious yet sometimes as serious. The pre-school child, particularly from $1-3\frac{1}{2}$ years, is vulnerable to separation from his mother. He is old enough to grieve over his loss, yet neither old enough to understand the reason nor to be comforted by others. The young child admitted to hospital may go through 3 stages (Fig. 1).

1 Protest, on the first day, as he cries for his mother and shouts for her return, perhaps standing up in the cot shaking the rails angrily.

2 Withdrawal, as he curls up in his cot quietly mourning over his loss. He refuses to eat or play with others, but may get some comfort from a dummy or favourite cuddly bit of material. The mourning phase can last for many days.

3 Denial—of the memory of his mother. He is superficially happy, making quick casual friendships with everyone, holding hands with and kissing the doctors and nurses. By this stage the mother–child relationship has been damaged, and when the child goes home a new bond will have to be fashioned. Meanwhile, there will be tantrums, nightmares, food refusal, bed wetting and other behaviour problems.

Prolonged separation may produce prolonged harm including physical and emotional illness in later life, delinquency and unstable marriages. Therefore management of the ill child, particularly those pre-school children who are most vulnerable to mother–child separation, involves:

1 Avoiding hospital admission unless it is essential.

2 Reducing the length of any admission to a minimum. The child is sent home still ill if there is no need for special hospital investigation or care. Many operations and procedures are done as 'day cases', the child being admitted, operated upon and sent home within 9 hours so that overnight stay is not needed.

3 Encouraging parents to visit their ill child in hospital at any time (unrestricted visiting), and creating facilities for mothers to sleep in hospital with their child.

For those children who have to be in hospital there is much that can be done to reduce the stress. Children are grouped together so that they may be looked after by qualified staff specially trained in the care of children. This segregation from adults also allows the children's wards to be made more homely. Good children's wards give an impression more of happy chaos than of highly organized medical technology (which is in fact going on). Teachers and play leaders are used to organize education and play and nurse allocation tries to ensure that each child is able to identify with one or two particular nurses.

MANAGEMENT

The child

An important part of the doctor's role is to anticipate and prevent needless pain or anxiety for the child. All children dislike 'pricks' whether they be venepunctures or intramuscular injections. Some are necessary but they must be kept to a minimum. Children respect and require honesty. It is wrong to say that painful procedures don't hurt; the child later feels tricked and trust is lost. Nevertheless, suggestion plays a part in most things so it is fair to minimize the pain—'it will hurt a little, just at the beginning, but not a lot'. Strange apparatus should be kept out of sight until it is used, then it must be explained, 'the X-ray machine is held up by a very strong metal rope which cannot break—it takes a photograph and does not hurt'.

The parents

The mother of an ill child tends to be labelled either 'an anxious mum' or 'a careless parent'. The land between, in which the parents show what most doctors and nurses consider 'reasonable' concern, is scanty and rarely inhabited. The doctor dealing with anxious parents needs compassion, tact and skill to help them.

Parental guilt at the time of a child's illness is common—they may have brought a weak congenitally handicapped child into the world, there may have been an accident involving the child for which they feel negligent, or an illness which they think would not have happened if they had 'given more vitamins', or

6

'kept her out of the rain'. These worries need to be ventilated and the doctor's role is that of listener and helper. The guilt feelings and the widespread feeling of inferiority to doctors and nurses make communication difficult, therefore the doctor must actively encourage them to talk, and anticipate their problems.

Because the general level of the parents' medical information may be 30 years out of date, their worries may be unsuspected by sophisticated medical and nursing staff. They may think that vomiting means something wrong with the abdomen, not knowing that it is a common feature of most febrile illnesses of childhood. They will worry if their child is not eating—almost as if he will perish from starvation, and therefore they need to be told that an ill child can manage well on drinks alone for a few days. It is worth remembering that the press and television tend to create topical diseases, and that parents may be worrying about rare conditions such as autism or leukaemia because of recent publicity.

Parents worry needlessly about rare diseases because they see tests done which are neither explained nor reported to them. They fear leukaemia because of a routine blood test. The level of explanation varies with each family. The language must be relevant to that family, and like all important messages must be repeated on another occasion. Many parents may want to know the name of the child's illness, but all parents want to know how it will affect the child. Similarly they are more concerned about what the surgeon *did* than what the child *had*. The days of the omniscient doctor are on the decline. Most parents want a kind and conscientious human being to help their child rather than a mystical god.

It is honest and respectable to admit: 'I don't know what the matter is' provided that one goes on to say 'but I do know what we must do to find out and to help.'

Episodes of illness should leave the parents more confident and not less. Doctors and nurses must beware of taking over the child and leaving the parents without a role and without self respect. There are always things a parent can do, and will do better than us, and we should say so. 'Please will you put on his nappy, you'll do it better than me'. However poor the mother is at mothering there will always be something we can find to praise in her care. This we must do—she is the only mother that

7

child will ever have, and she is the best that the child will ever have. In our dealings with her we must make sure she emerges proud, confident, and competent with her child.

Further reading

Apley J. & MacKeith R.C. (1968) *The Child and his Symptoms*, Chapters 23–26. Blackwell Scientific Publications, Oxford.

Chapter 2

THE NEWBORN BABY

It is essential that all doctors should be capable of making a competent examination of newborn babies, of recognizing ill health and congenital defect at the earliest possible moment, and of dealing with those problems which demand immediate action. The **examination of the infant immediately after birth** is most commonly carried out by the midwife and is usually confined to determining (a) that there is nothing to interfere with the establishment of normal respiration, and (b) that there are no gross external deformities. Within the first 24–48 hours of life every baby should be examined in detail by a doctor. Naturally, if the baby shows any evidence of ill health before this time, thorough examination is needed immediately. At no other time of life does illness, or suspicion of illness, demand such urgent attention. Delay, even of a few minutes, may have disastrous consequences. It is for this reason that all low birth weight babies, ill babies, and others requiring any special attention in a maternity unit are gathered together in a special care baby unit, where medical and nursing staff with experience of newborns are constantly available.

The **routine examination** of the apparently healthy baby is intended to assess his general health and to diagnose promptly congenital anomalies, especially those which require urgent treatment. The examination will be most satisfactory if it is carried out when the baby is awake but contented, a happy frame of mind most likely to be encountered shortly after a feed. His general health can best be judged without disturbing him by observing his colour, the posture in which he lies, the way he moves, and (if he cries) by the nature of his cry. Examination of muscle tone is also informative, but can often be inferred from observations of posture and movement. The normal colour,

9

posture and cry cannot be described: they can be learned from newborn babies.

Some important observations made routinely by the midwife will also help the doctor to assess the baby's health. These include measurement of weight, length and head circumference, and observation of urine and meconium, both of which are usually

Table 1. Routine Examination of Newborn Infant

Examination	Conditions sought
Skin and subcutaneous fat	Intra-uterine malnutrition
Head circumference, sutures, fontanelles	Hydrocephalus
Facial features and pinnae	Malformation syndromes (e.g. mongolism) Facial palsy
Eyes	Glaucoma: cataract: corneal opacities
Mouth	Cleft palate: congenital teeth
Jaw	Abnormal size or position of mandible
Chest	Abnormalities of lungs
Heart	Congenital heart disease: mediastinal displacement
Abdomen	Abnormal masses (e.g. cystic kidneys)
Perineum	Genital anomalies: anal anomalies
Hips	Instability or dislocation
Femoral pulses	Coarctation of aorta
Back	Spina bifida: dermal sinus: post-anal dimple
Limbs	Talipes: abnormal long bones and digits: palmar creases
Reflexes and responses (sucking, swallowing, Moro)	Maturity of central nervous system

passed within 24 hours of birth. Meconium changes to milk stools on days 3–4. The umbilical cord has usually separated by 7 days but may take a few days longer.

The routine examination of the newborn baby should include attention to the points listed in Table 1. Such examination will reveal most, but not all, defects. Congenital heart disease especially may not be detectable for days or weeks. Renal tract anomalies, unless gross, are not detected until urinary infection supervenes and points the need for pyelography. Metabolic disease may need to be sought by biochemical testing, either on a population basis, as in screening for phenylketonuria, or in selected infants if there is a relevant family history.

CONGENITAL MALFORMATIONS

About 2% of all babies are born with serious congenital defects, sufficient to threaten life, to cause permanent handicap, or to require surgical correction. Malformations therefore form a major cause of perinatal and infant death, and constitute one of the greatest problems in paediatrics. Defects of the central nervous system and heart account for more than half the total. Most of the common defects are described in the relevant chapters: here some general principles will be considered.

Distressingly little is known of the causes of congenital abnormalities. Single gene defects and chromosome anomalies account for 10–20% of the total. A small number are attributable to rubella, and fewer to teratogenic drugs and ionizing radiation. The causes of most common defects remain unknown, although some aetiological factors are known. For example, some defects are more common in certain ethnic groups, socio-economic groups, or at some maternal ages and parities than others. It is believed that most non-genetic defects arise from the simultaneous action of many adverse factors upon a susceptible embryo.

The incidence of serious defects and chromosomal anomalies amongst early spontaneous abortuses is very high. Nature has devised a fairly efficient system for terminating at the first possible moment pregnancies which are doomed to failure. It can be shown, for example, that at least 90% of mongols and a much higher proportion of embryos with sex chromosome anomalies are aborted. Live-born, malformed infants therefore represent the small minority for which this mechanism has failed.

Early diagnosis of congenital anomalies is necessary because:
1 it may influence the management of pregnancy and delivery;
2 prompt treatment may be necessary;
3 parents need early information and advice.

Major anomalies can sometimes be diagnosed before birth.

The development of polyhydramnios (excess amniotic fluid) in a pregnant woman will always prompt an abdominal X-ray. This may show twins, or an anencephalic fetus, in which the cerebral hemispheres and cranial vault are absent. Hydrocephalus may also be diagnosed by X-ray, and occasionally the bony anomalies of spina bifida may be seen. In recent years newer techniques of prenatal diagnosis have opened up exciting possibilities. Ultrasound provides a means of measuring fetal skull size—thereby monitoring fetal growth as well as diagnosing twins and anencephaly. Cells from amniotic fluid samples (obtainable by amniocentesis from about 14 weeks) are of fetal origin. They can be cultured and karyotyped, permitting, for example, the diagnosis of mongolism, or examined for enzyme defects which allows many serious metabolic disorders to be recognized. Levels of alpha-fetoprotein in amniotic fluid are consistently raised if the fetus has anencephaly or open myelomeningocele. These techniques are at present applied to high-risk mothers with a view to selective abortion, but screening of all pregnant mothers could lead to the virtual disappearance of mongolism and spina bifida.

Most congenital defects will be revealed by the careful clinical examination already described. Others can only be suspected when they give rise to symptoms such as vomiting, cyanosis, jaundice, or failure to pass urine or meconium. When a congenital defect has been firmly diagnosed, the information has to be given to the parents together with an indication of the prognosis.

The news that a baby is deformed is a great shock to the parents. Even minor anomalies are seen as major tragedies. At the first interview detailed explanations will not be grasped. If the baby is to be transferred to another hospital for early surgery, the mother must have a chance to see her infant before removal. She will need frequent progress reports on the baby until she is able to visit. The closer the contact the parents maintain with the baby, the less likely are they to reject it if there is a residual handicap. If the baby survives, the parents need patient explanation of the care needed and how to recognize any problems that are likely to arise. They will almost certainly feel that the infant's deformity is somehow their fault, and will wonder why it happened to them. They will need advice about the recurrence risks if they plan another child later on. All this implies ready access to doctors and nurses who can listen and answer, and who can at least give the appearance of having unlimited time to spare. Parents of seriously handicapped children can often help one another through membership of parents' associations or organizations. Such associations exist not only for the parents of children with serious malformations such as spina bifida, but also for those with mental handicap, cerebral palsy, muscular dystrophy, cystic fibrosis, leukaemia, infantile autism, deafness and blindness, and coeliac disease.

In summary, whenever a malformed baby is born the parents want to know:

1   exactly what is the matter, in terms they can grasp;
2   what can the doctors do about it;
3   what can the parents do about it;
4   what is the outlook for this child;
5   what is the outlook for any other children that may follow;
6   finally, parents want to know why it happened, but only exceptionally can this be answered.

PERINATAL ASPHYXIA

Before birth the fetus is dependent for his oxygen supply upon (a) a normal oxygen tension in the mother's blood; (b) a healthy placenta firmly attached to the uterine wall; and (c) unobstructed blood flow through the umbilical vessels. After birth, the newborn baby's oxygenation depends upon (a) a functioning respiratory centre; (b) a patent airway; and (c) healthy heart and lungs. Interference with one or more of these functions is likely to lead to hypoxia, either before birth or immediately afterwards (see Fig. 2). Hypoxia before birth is recognized by the signs of fetal distress of which the most important are bradycardia and meconium staining of the liquor. These signs are not very reliable, and more direct evidence of hypoxia and acidosis is now being sought by estimations of pO_2 and pH on blood samples obtained from the fetal scalp when the cervix is sufficiently widely dilated. After birth, hypoxia is recognized by alterations of pulse, respiration, colour, tone and reflex irritability, the last being tested either by slapping the feet or inserting a catheter into the nares. It is now almost universal practice to score these 5 attributes on a

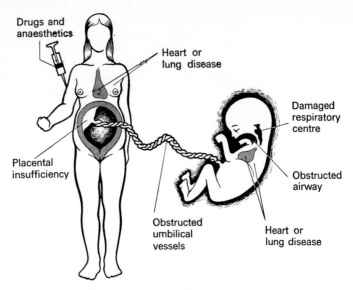

Fig. 2. Causes of asphyxia neonatorum.

0,1,2 scale, the total score ranging from 0 for a dead baby to 10 for one in the pink of condition. This is the *Apgar score*, named after the late Dr Virginia Apgar who described the method. Details are shown in Table 2. The score is normally assessed one minute after birth, and at 5 and 10 minutes if necessary. A score

Table 2. Apgar Score

Sign	0	1	2
Heart rate	Absent	Below 100/min	100/min or higher
Respiratory effort	Nil	Slow, irregular	Regular, with cry
Muscle tone	Limp	Some tone in limbs	Active movements
Reflex irritability	Nil	Grimace only	Cry
Colour	Pallor or generalized cyanosis	Body pink, extremities blue	Pink all over

of 7 or higher is satisfactory and no intervention is called for. A score of 3 or less indicates severe hypoxia and impending death.

It will be seen in Table 3 that hypoxia, by damaging the respiratory centre, may cause further hypoxia. This downhill spiral can only be reversed by improving the oxygen supply to the brain before the circulation stops, the most efficient method being endotracheal intubation and positive pressure insufflation. Apgar scores in the intermediate range of 4–6 usually indicate

Table 3. Perinatal Oxygen Supply

Requirements	Potential Threats
A. *Before Birth*	
Normal oxygen tension in mother's blood	Advanced heart or lung disease
	Unskilled anaesthesia
Healthy placenta, firmly attached	Placental insufficiency
	Placental abruption ⎫ (premature
	⎬ separation of
	Placenta praevia ⎭ the placenta)
Unobstructed umbilical vessels	Prolapsed cord
	Ruptured cord; knotted cord
	Prolonged labour
B. *At Birth*	
Functioning respiratory centre	Intracranial haemorrhage
	Cerebral hypoxia
	Respiratory depressant drugs
Patent airway	Mucus, blood, meconium in airway
	Retrognathia (jaw too far back)
	Micrognathia (jaw too small)
	Choanal atresia (blocked nasopharynx)
Healthy heart and lungs	Diaphragmatic hernia
	Major anomalies of the lungs
	Severe congenital heart lesions

the need for simple measures, including clearing of the airway by suction, gentle stimulation of the baby, and the administration of oxygen by face mask. Nalorphine hydrobromide should be given, 1 mg i.v. or i.m. if the mother has been given pethidine or morphine derivatives during labour.

The fetus deprived of oxygen responds initially by increased respiratory effort. If this is unavailing, respiration becomes more and more feeble and then stops (primary apnoea). After a short time respiration begins again and continues until the last gasp, which is followed by secondary (terminal) apnoea. Failure to distinguish between primary and secondary apnoea has led to some of the confusion about the efficacy of resuscitative measures.

Newborn babies are capable of utilizing some anaerobic metabolic pathways and can therefore tolerate hypoxia of more severe degree than can older children or adults. Nevertheless, the condition is serious and requires urgent and skilled attention because the brain is the tissue most sensitive to oxygen lack, and severe hypoxia may cause death, mental defect, cerebral palsy or other permanent neurological disorders. In general, a baby who establishes regular respiration within 10 minutes of birth will probably develop normally: after 20 minutes the outlook is less certain: and if respiration has not been established after 30 minutes the outlook is very grim. Neonatal convulsions following hypoxia are a bad prognostic sign.

BIRTH INJURY

The term birth injury is usually used in respect of physical injury, as distinct from the chemical injury of hypoxia, hyper-bilirubinaemia and hypoglycaemia. The distinction between intracranial birth injury and hypoxia is not clear, since hypoxia can cause capillary damage leading to intraventricular haemorrhage, and the haemorrhage resulting from tears of the falx cerebri or tentorium cerebelli may damage the respiratory centre and lead to hypoxia. Intracranial birth injury may occur if the baby is very small (with soft skull and brain) or very large (with consequent mechanical problems); if labour is very rapid, causing rapid compression and decompression of the head; if there is malpresentation of the fetus; or if there is difficult forceps delivery. These may cause intracerebral, subarachnoid or sub-dural haemorrhage, leading to death or survival with brain damage. Nothing can be done directly to stop bleeding. Treatment is as for severe hypoxia but is often unavailing.

Skull fracture

Skull fracture is not uncommon but is usually linear without displacement, causing no symptoms and needing no treatment.

A localized, depressed fracture is usually best treated by elevation of the bone, although if there are no focal signs it may heal without sequelae.

Cephalhaematoma

Cephalhaematoma results from bleeding between a skull bone and the overlying periosteum. One or both parietals are commonly affected, the occipital occasionally, the frontals never. The swelling is soft and fluctuant and conforms in shape and position to a cranial bone (Fig. 3). It cannot cross a suture. Some resolve within a few weeks: others calcify, especially around the periphery, and take longer to go. In neither case is any treatment required, beyond explanation and reassurance to the parents.

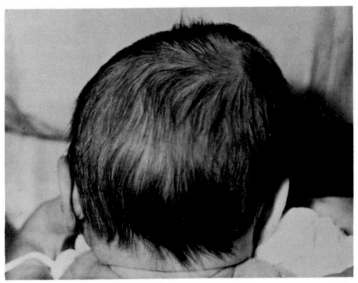

Fig. 3. Cephalhaematoma of the right parietal region.

Sub-aponeurotic haemorrhage

This disorder is rare but serious. It may occur in babies with blood clotting defects (e.g. Factor V deficiency). The bleeding occurs into the 'scalping' layer and spreads over the whole surface of the vault of the skull. As the newborn's total blood volume is about 300 ml, he can easily bleed to death into the sub-aponeurotic layer. Rapid recognition, prompt transfusion, and the correction of any clotting defect will save lives.

Apart from the skull, fractures are only likely to arise when there is difficulty delivering the infant's shoulders, when the bones likely to break are the clavicle and the humerus. These fractures always unite without deformity.

Nerve palsies

The same shoulder-stretching force may injure the brachial plexus and cause nerve palsies. The more common Erb's palsy results from stretching of the upper roots of the plexus. The arm lies straight and limp beside the body, internally rotated and with the fingers flexed (usually referred to as the waiter's tip, or in shadier parts the policeman's tip, position, but probably only seen in these gentlemen if they have brachial plexus lesions). The far less common paralysis of the hand seen after injury to the lower cords of the plexus is named after Klumpke, who described it when she was a medical student. In the great majority of cases the injury causes physiological rather than anatomical interruption of nerve conduction, and spontaneous recovery occurs.

The only other common nerve injury in the newborn is facial palsy. It is a lower motor neurone defect, usually unilateral. It may be associated with, and attributed to, the use of forceps but can occur without. Recovery is the rule.

LOW BIRTH WEIGHT

Babies of low birth weight have special problems and need special care. Recent changes in terminology are potentially confusing and warrant explanation. For many years the term 'prematurity' was used to describe babies with birthweights of 2500 g ($5\frac{1}{2}$ lb) or less, most of whom were born after gestation periods of 36 weeks or less. However, birth weight and length of gestation do not always march hand in hand. One baby may weigh less than 2500 g at full term, while a diabetic mother may be delivered at 36 weeks of an infant weighing 4000 g or more. 'Maturity' is a concept which means different things to different people and is not susceptible to precise measurement. Birth weight can be measured accurately and length of gestation reliably in most cases. Babies may be born of low birth weight *either* because their gestation period was cut short, *or* because their intra-uterine growth has been retarded. In some infants, both factors operate. We can therefore define two groups of babies requiring special care (Fig. 4).

1   Pre-term babies (less than 37 weeks' gestation). Most will be of low birth weight, but the babies of diabetic and prediabetic mothers, however large, face the same problems.

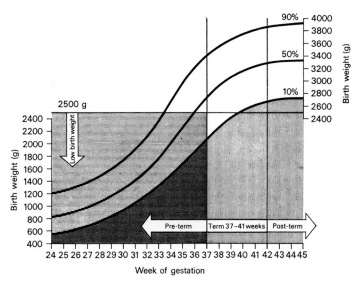

Fig. 4. Pre-term babies (horizontal hatching) are of less than 37 weeks gestation. Light-for-dates babies (vertical hatching) have a weight below the 10% for their gestation.

2   Light-for-dates babies (birth weight inappropriately low in relation to the length of gestation).

The length of gestation is normally calculated from the first day of the mother's last period and from serial observations of fundal height. In cases of doubt, the development of fetal epiphyses may be studied on X-rays, but correlate better with fetal size than with length of gestation. The biparietal diameter of the fetal skull estimated by ultrasound correlates well with gestation. Experimentally, a number of biochemical, cytochemical and cytological tests on amniotic fluid are being developed, which may be helpful in selected cases.

At birth the gestational age of the baby may be estimated from weight, length and head circumference; from certain physical characteristics; by the maturity of the nervous system as assessed by eliciting various reflexes and responses; and in special cases by assessing biochemical maturity in terms of, for example, immunoglobulins or haemoglobins.

The use of the term 'dysmaturity' to describe certain clinical features exhibited by many light-for-dates babies is discouraged, but will remain in use until a satisfactory alternative has been invented. These features include a lack of subcutaneous fat and dry, wrinkled or cracked skin. 'Postmaturity' should be used, if at all, to mean an excessively long gestation period. 'Placental insufficiency' can only be diagnosed on the basis of placental function tests, of which the most generally used is the maternal urinary excretion of oestriol. Levels which fall, or rise too slowly, with advancing pregnancy strongly suggest impaired placental function.

Pre-term baby (Fig. 5)

The main problems are:
1 feeding;
2 hyperbilirubinaemia;
3 respiratory distress syndrome;
4 infections;
5 brain damage;
6 anaemia and vitamin deficiency.

The special problems of *feeding* premature babies arise from:
i   their poorly developed sucking and swallowing reflexes;
ii   the ease with which they regurgitate feeds and may inhale milk, with a risk of inhalation pneumonia;
iii their large calorie requirement in relation to size.

If sucking and swallowing reflexes are inadequate, or if bottle feeding causes the baby to become exhausted, feeds will be given by gastric tube. The risk of regurgitation is minimized by giving small, frequent feeds and reducing the handling of the infant to

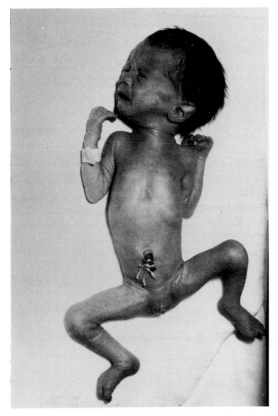

Fig. 5. A pre-term baby of 34 weeks gestation. She is jaundiced, has prominent labia minora and is lying in a characteristic 'frog's legs' position.

a minimum. However, to provide adequate calories, the size of the feeds must be increased as rapidly as the infant will tolerate them. Satisfactory weight gain may not be achieved until the infant is receiving as much as 150 cal/kg/day.

Jaundice

Jaundice occurs in all pre-term babies: the more immature the baby, the more marked is the jaundice. This is because the liver enzyme glucuronyl transferase, which is required for the conjugation of bilirubin prior to its excretion, is poorly developed in the newborn, and especially in the pre-term baby. Occasionally bilirubin levels may become dangerously high (250–350 μmol/l or more) with the threat of kernicterus, and exchange transfusion is required. This is more likely to occur if the baby has been hypoxic at any stage or if feeding has been delayed.

The idiopathic respiratory distress syndrome

Sometimes called hyaline membrane disease, idiopathic respiratory distress syndrome is a dangerous illness seen only in the newborn period and confined almost entirely to pre-term babies. Affected babies may breathe reasonably well at birth and to the untrained eye may appear to be healthy. Respiration is, however, a little laboured, and becomes progressively more so with the passage of time. Over the course of a few hours respiratory effort increases, but with diminishing effect. With each breath, instead of the lungs expanding, the soft parts of the chest wall sink in so that there is visible recession of the intercostal spaces, the suprasternal fossa and the epigastrium. There may be an audible grunt, and the baby's colour deteriorates. In severe cases there is cyanosis and cardiac failure. Biochemical studies show a profound acidosis, part respiratory and part metabolic, lowered pO_2 and raised pCO_2. The condition proceeds either to death or to complete recovery: sequelae are rare. A chest X-ray shows a granular appearance over the whole of the lungfields. In fatal cases, histological examination of the lungs usually shows an eosinophilic material lining the alveoli and terminal bronchioles (hyaline membrane) which consists largely of fibrin. Chemical examination of the lung fluid shows a marked depletion of surfactant, a lipoprotein normally present in lung fluid and having the property of lowering surface tension and preventing adhesion of alveolar walls. Treatment includes the administration of oxygen, the correction of acidosis by administering intravenous sodium bicarbonate in carefully calculated amounts, the maintenance of calorie intake, and the control of cardiac failure. If respiratory insufficiency is severe and prolonged, assisted ventilation is indicated, but the mortality rate in severe cases remains around 30–50%.

Estimation of the lipid content of amniotic fluid (lecithin and sphyngomyelin) provides a good guide to the development of surfactant and the risk of respiratory distress. When early induction of labour is planned, this test can help in deciding the best time for the baby.

Respiratory distress may also occur in pneumonia, with pulmonary haemorrhage and in babies with brain damage.

Infections

The liability of the pre-term infant to infections is largely determined by the immaturity of his humoral immunity. The greatest risk is from gram-negative bacterial infections, especially pneumonia, septicaemia and meningitis. An additional risk stems from the difficulty of recognizing such infections when they arise. The usual signs of infection, both clinical and laboratory, seen in older children or adults may be entirely absent, and the first clue to trouble may be poor feeding, regurgitation, jaundice, unexplained weight loss, or a slight rise or fall of body temperature. In no area of medicine does more depend upon accurate observation and records, and the watchful eye of an experienced nurse. Chest X-rays, blood cultures and lumbar punctures may need to be done on little more than a suspicion of trouble. Once the diagnosis is obvious, it is almost certainly too late for effective treatment.

Brain damage

The pre-term brain is a very soft organ, almost fluid, and the blood vessels within and around it have very delicate walls. The forces to which the fetal skull and its contents are exposed in normal labour may be sufficient to cause brain damage in the small baby: difficult labour is even more hazardous. The obstetrician minimizes the trauma by carrying out episiotomy and delivering the baby with extra care. Risks to the brain after birth include hyperbilirubinaemia, hypoglycaemia and meningitis. Earlier follow-up studies of pre-term babies, especially those of very low birth weight, revealed a depressingly high incidence of physical and mental defect. More recent studies from modern neonatal units providing comprehensive monitoring, show more encouraging results, the incidence of handicap being scarcely greater than in full-term babies.

Anaemia

Pre-term babies often develop quite severe anaemia when 2 or 3 months old. The aetiology is complex. The anaemia can usually be prevented by giving prophylactic iron supplements, or will respond to iron if it has developed. The deficiency arises from the disparity between the iron intake and the very rapid rate of growth, with a correspondingly rapid increase in blood volume. Sometimes the anaemia is megaloblastic and responds to folic acid. In a few pre-term babies anaemia is evident much earlier and results from temporary marrow hypoplasia. The rapid rate of growth also renders pre-term babies more prone to vitamin-deficiency diseases. It is therefore advisable that all pre-term babies should be given supplements of vitamins as well as iron until their diets contain adequate amounts (6–9 months).

Light-for-dates baby (Fig. 6)

The special problems of the light-for-dates baby are:
1 hypoglycaemia;
2 skin infection;
3 poor post-natal growth.

Neonatal hypoglycaemia

This disorder has only been recognized as a hazard to the newborn in relatively recent years, and it is not yet clear how serious a danger it is. The normal blood glucose level in the newborn is low in comparison to older infants. Symptoms are rarely seen unless the level falls below 1.0 mmol/l. The first symptoms are irritability, pallor and reluctance with feeds. Frank twitching proceeding to generalized convulsions occurs later. There is a danger that hypoglycaemia may cause brain damage and it is therefore necessary to recognize and treat the condition as early as possible. On the least suspicion the blood glucose level should be checked. The Dextrostix test is designed for use with adults,

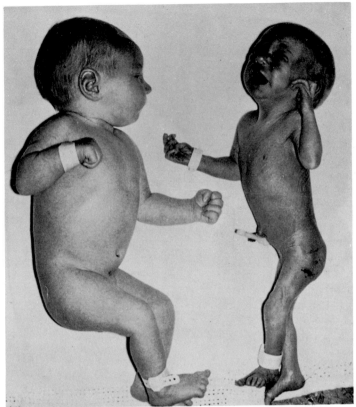

Fig. 6. Two babies born at 40 weeks gestation. That on the left weighs a normal 3.5 kg. That on the right is light-for-dates, weighing 2 kg; he is thin and has a dry wrinkled skin.

and the lowest normal colour reading represents glucose levels of 2.0 mmol/l or less. However, the very experienced eye can distinguish the colour difference between levels above and below 1.0 mmol/l, and a machine is now available which measures the depth of colour and is sufficiently delicate for use in the neonatal period. The best way to prevent neonatal hypoglycaemia is early feeding. Mild hypoglycaemia may be treated by frequent feeds with added glucose; more severe forms require intravenous glucose.

Skin infection

The dry, cracked skin of the light-for-dates baby renders it especially prone to skin infection with staphylococci. Infections are best treated by antiseptic creams.

Slow growth

Most light-for-dates babies are hungry and gain weight well. A few behave as if permanently adjusted to slow growth. They feed poorly from birth and appear to have small food requirements. They grow slowly, and their weight and height increase parallel to, but below, the 3rd centile on growth charts. Some of these infants have one or both parents well below average size. Bone age is usually retarded and epiphyses fuse relatively late, so there is an opportunity for some catch-up growth at puberty. As growth patterns are largely determined very early in life, every effort should be made to achieve good weight gain in the neonatal period.

JAUNDICE IN THE NEWBORN

Jaundice is extremely common in newborn infants and is usually noted on the 2nd or 3rd day of life, gradually fading over the next few days. This is *physiological jaundice* and results from a temporary inadequacy of supply of bilirubin glucuronyl transferase by the

Table 4.   Causes of Neonatal Jaundice

Type of jaundice	Causes
Bilirubin largely unconjugated	Physiological jaundice
	Haemolytic disease (Rhesus, ABO, etc.)
	Other haemolytic anaemias
	(hereditary spherocytosis: G6PD deficiency)
	After extensive internal bleeding
	(especially cephalhaematoma)
Bilirubin mixed	Sepsis (septicaemia or other severe infection)
	Neonatal hepatitis
	Galactosaemia
Bilirubin largely conjugated	Biliary atresia

liver. This is especially marked in pre-term babies virtually all of whom develop jaundice. Physiological jaundice may be protracted in cretins, and this may be the first diagnostic clue. In healthy, full-term babies bilirubin levels in physiological jaundice rarely exceed 200 μmol/l. In small, pre-term babies higher levels may be reached with the risk of kernicterus (p. 28). In these infants the administration of phenobarbitone, which acts as an enzyme inducer, or phototherapy with blue light, may prevent bilirubin levels becoming dangerously high, but exchange transfusion is sometimes needed.

Jaundice appearing in the first 24 hours of life is never physiological. It is more often due to haemolytic disease than to all other causes. Other causes of neonatal jaundice are shown in Table 4.

Haemolytic disease of the newborn

A woman may become sensitized to red cell antigens either as a result of fetal red cells leaking across the placental barrier, usually at the end of a pregnancy, or as a consequence of the transfusion of improperly matched blood. If, in her next pregnancy, the fetus has the same red cell antigen, maternal antibody will cross the placenta and begin to destroy fetal red cells. This is haemolytic disease, and most commonly occurs in a rhesus positive infant whose rhesus negative mother has become sensitized to the D rhesus antigen. Less commonly, haemolytic disease results from incompatibility of other rhesus antigens, ABO antigens, or the rare blood group antigens. Haemolysis leads to anaemia, the severity of which depends upon the rate of red cell destruction and the efficiency with which new red cells are produced. There is very active erythropoiesis in the liver and spleen as well as in the marrow, and primitive red cells—reticulocytes, normoblasts, erythroblasts—are plentiful in the peripheral blood: hence the alternative name, erythroblastosis fetalis. In the most severe cases, the profound anaemia leads to fetal heart failure with gross oedema (hydrops fetalis) which carries a very high mortality rate.

Bilirubin conjugation and excretion are carried on fairly efficiently by the fetus in utero. The amniotic fluid is bile-stained, but the serum bilirubin level of cord blood is never more than

27

100 μmol/l unless there is an element of obstructive jaundice (inspissated bile syndrome). After birth, however, the bilirubin level begins to climb and clinical jaundice becomes evident or more marked within a few hours of birth. Haemolytic disease is by far the most common cause of jaundice noticed within 24 hours of birth in Caucasian infants. Because of the relative inefficiency of the neonatal liver, especially in pre-term babies, the serum bilirubin level may reach 350–500 μmol/l or more. This is predominantly unconjugated bilirubin, which is soluble in lipid but not in water. If the level is allowed to rise too high, bilirubin may be deposited in the grey matter of the brain, especially the basal ganglia, causing kernicterus. This is the most dangerous complication of haemolytic disease, leading to death or to survival with permanent brain damage. Clinically, it presents with irritability, poor feeding, head retraction, down-turned eyes ('setting sun sign') and convulsions. Late sequelae include mental defect, cerebral palsy (athetoid or spastic) and perceptive deafness.

Haemolytic disease is now preventable unless the mother has already developed antibodies. The initial sensitizing event virtually always occurs around the time of birth of a rhesus positive baby. If anti-D immunoglobulin is given to all rhesus negative women by intravenous injection shortly after delivery, any D positive cells in her circulation (fetal cells) will be destroyed before the mother has begun to develop any antibodies to them. Any remaining injected antibody is eliminated very quickly. At present there is no shortage of anti-D immunoglobulin from the blood of women who have developed rhesus antibodies. As the number of such women is gradually reduced towards zero, it may be necessary to sensitize rhesus negative male volunteers.

For those women who already have antibodies, prevention is not possible. All their rhesus positive babies will be affected. The clinical picture at birth varies from the mildest with no abnormal signs, through moderate with definite pallor and some enlargement of the liver and spleen, to severe with profound anaemia, marked hepatosplenomegaly and perhaps jaundice. The direct Coombs' test is positive, and the haemoglobin and bilirubin levels in cord blood give a useful indication of the severity of the disease. Mildly affected infants require no treatment at birth. The haemoglobin will fall over the next 6–8 weeks; if it drops below 7g/dL, simple transfusion is advisable. More severe cases require transfusion earlier and perhaps more than once. The most severe cases, as judged by clinical and laboratory findings, and in the light of the history of previously affected children, may require exchange transfusion. This procedure replaces most of the infant's blood with donor rhesus negative blood (which will not be destroyed by antibody), raises the haemoglobin level, and removes most of the doomed rhesus positive cells together with some circulating bilirubin. In a few infants more than one exchange transfusion may be necessary.

A severely affected infant may not survive to full term, and a decision may have to be made to deliver the infant earlier. The hazards of immaturity are then added to those of haemolytic disease, and the decision calls for experience and judgement. It is based upon the previous history and examination of liquor amnii. Affected infants tend to be at least as severely affected as the previous child. The concentration of bilirubin in amniotic fluid generally reflects the severity of the disease. The titre of rhesus antibody in the mother's blood can be estimated, but is not such a reliable guide.

Only haemolytic disease due to D antigen will be anticipated by routine antenatal blood tests. The remaining cases will only be recognized when an infant develops jaundice within 24 hours of birth. ABO incompatibility most commonly occurs in a group A baby of a group O mother. It is usually mild. Rare blood group incompatibilities can only be diagnosed by special haematological investigation, and it may be difficult to find suitable donor blood for exchange transfusion.

OTHER NEONATAL PROBLEMS

Haemorrhagic disease of the newborn

Just as the liver of the newborn baby, and especially of the pre-term baby, takes a few days to become competent at conjugating bilirubin, so it is temporarily inefficient at synthesizing many blood clotting factors. Serial measurements of the prothrombin level, for example, will usually show a fall from cord blood levels until about the third day of life, after which it improves, reaching normal levels about 7–10 days after birth. In the great majority of infants there are no clinical symptoms, but occasionally there is spontaneous bleeding, usually from the gastrointestinal tract, on the 2nd or 3rd day of life. Melaena is recognizable by a dark red tinge to the meconium; vomited blood is usually dark brown. The amount of blood lost is rarely enough to disturb health, but occasionally there is sufficient blood loss to necessitate transfusion. Otherwise treatment comprises the intramuscular injection of Vitamin K_1, 1 mg, repeated if necessary.

Pre-term and anoxic infants are more prone to develop haemorrhagic disease than healthy, full-term babies. Prophylactic Vitamin K_1 may be given at birth to infants at particular risk, but some paediatricians prefer every infant to receive it.

Deficiency of clotting factors may also contribute to bleeding from the umbilicus or into the subaponeurotic space of the scalp. The latter is much more serious than cephalhaematoma (p. 17), because the extent of the bleeding is almost unlimited and the baby may become exsanguinated with alarming rapidity. Other causes of neonatal gastrointestinal bleeding include:

1 Swallowed maternal blood, either
   (a) following antepartum or intrapartum haemorrhage, or
   (b) as a result of feeding from engorged breasts.
Large amounts of blood may be vomited, but the baby shows no signs of blood loss. If the blood has not become denatured in the stomach, maternal blood can be distinguished chemically from infant's blood.

2 Hiatus hernia. The predominant feature is vomiting; there may be a little altered blood, but frank melaena is rare.

Infections

Some babies are born infected, some acquire infection during birth, and some have infection thrust upon them after birth. The principal infections in each category are as follows:

1 Acquired before birth:
   (a) syphilis,
   (b) rubella,
   (c) toxoplasmosis,
   (d) cytomegalovirus infection.

2 Acquired during birth:
   (a) gonorrhoea,
   (b) moniliasis.
3 Acquired after birth:
   (a) staphylococcal infections of the skin, umbilicus, eye or nail-bed,
   (b) gram-negative bacterial infections (commonly *E. coli*)—septicaemia, meningitis, pneumonia, urinary tract infections.

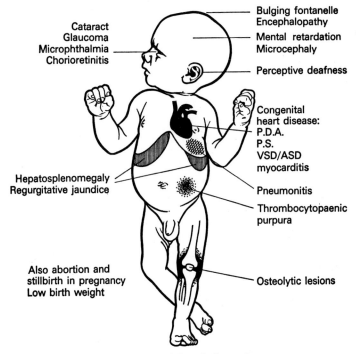

Fig. 7. Features of the rubella syndrome.

Infection of a developing embryo is likely to cause death and abortion. The *rubella* virus, although undoubtedly capable of causing embryonic death, also has the unique ability to cause malformations compatible with life, notably congenital heart disease, cataract and other eye defects, perceptive deafness, and microcephaly with mental retardation. In addition, an infected baby may be born with evidence of active viraemia as shown by jaundice, hepatosplenomegaly, purpura and sometimes lesions of the bones and lungs (Fig. 7). This 'extended rubella syndrome' can occur without malformations. A baby with congenital rubella has persisting endogenous antibody and may also excrete live virus from the pharynx and the kidneys for as long as 2 years. Congenital rubella may be confirmed by isolation of virus from throat washings or urine, by demonstrating specific rubella IgM in the baby, or by persistence of rubella antibody after the age of 8 months.

Hepatitis is a conspicuous feature of other intrauterine infections, the liver being the first organ reached by blood from the placenta. Jaundice and hepatomegaly are therefore common presenting features. In *congenital syphilis*, which is very rare in Britain now, skin rashes and snuffles may be present at birth. Infection with *Toxoplasma gondii* or *cytomegalovirus* may damage the central nervous system or eye, resulting in mental retardation, epilepsy, microcephaly, hydrocephalus, microphthalmia or choroiditis. These diagnoses are confirmed by serological tests on infant and mother.

The common '*sticky eye*' is essentially a drainage problem. If tears cannot drain adequately down the naso-lacrymal duct they tend to pool in the inner canthus in the supine infant. In this pool the ubiquitous staphylococcus multiplies, producing a small amount of pus which dries. The conjunctivae remain clear. The condition subsides within 2–3 weeks. Secretions can be gently bathed away as necessary: antibiotics, though often used, are only necessary in severe cases. By contrast, *gonococcal ophthalmia*, which was once the commonest cause of blindness in children, is now rare. There is much periorbital oedema which makes it difficult to open the eyes. If the lids are forced apart, copious, creamy, pale yellow pus wells out. Vigorous treatment is needed with an antibiotic to which the organism is sensitive.

Oral thrush (moniliasis) present within a few days of birth is often the result of a maternal infection of the genital tract. If the infection develops later, it is more likely to have been acquired from unsterilized dummies, teats or bottles. The source of infection should be traced if possible and dealt with by treatment or advice. Nystatin suspension should be applied to the mouth lesions after feeds. Monilial infections in other sites are rare in the newborn period.

E. Coli is the most dangerous organism to the newborn baby. It may cause septicaemia, meningitis, pneumonia, urinary infection or gastro-enteritis. It can probably be acquired either during or after birth and is responsible for most of the serious and lethal infections of the neonate. Whereas the alimentary tract of the breast fed baby is colonised by lactobacilli, in the bottle-fed baby *E. coli* is predominant. The early signs of infection in the newborn are inconspicuous and will only be detected by the experienced and vigilant eye. A reluctance to feed, a slightly loose stool, slight vomiting, unsatisfactory weight gain, a cyanotic attack, irritability or a small flick of temperature may be the first hint of trouble. Later, vomiting, diarrhoea, weight loss, fever, convulsions, jaundice or rash make it obvious that the baby is ill. There is often little in the way of localizing symptoms or signs. Blood culture, lumbar puncture, chest X-ray and urine examination will be needed, but if clinical suspicions exist, parenteral antibiotics must be started without waiting for laboratory reports. The longer the delay, the greater the risk of death or brain damage. Amongst the many antibiotic regimes advocated, penicillin *or* ampicillin together with gentamicin are widely used.

Staphylococcal infections are very common but rarely severe. Sticky eyes, septic spots, sticky umbilicus and paronychia will respond to simple local measures. More severe skin infections require systemic antibiotics (e.g. cloxacillin).

Hypocalcaemia

Hypocalcaemic tetany characteristically occurs in bottle-fed babies about a week old. It presents with localized twitchings, especially of the hands and feet, or with generalized convulsions. The serum calcium is usually below 1.8 μmol/l, and this may be partly due to the high phosphate content of cow's milk in comparison with human milk. Mild cases are treated with oral calcium supplements and sedation, more severe cases with parenteral calcium. The convulsions usually respond readily and the long-term prognosis is good. Less frequently hypocalcaemia arises in the first 3 days of life: the reason for this is obscure.

Occasionally hypocalcaemia fails to respond to adequate doses of calcium. It may then be found that the serum magnesium is below the normal 0.5–1 μmol/l. Intramuscular magnesium sulphate is effective treatment. Hypomagnesaemia without hypocalcaemia is excessively rare.

Convulsions

Convulsions are always a serious symptom and nowhere more so than in the neonatal period. The cause must be determined and, if possible, treated. Most fits will respond to phenobarbitone or chloral hydrate unless there is severe brain damage. The main causes of neonatal convulsions have been described in this chapter, and are summarized below.

1 Brain damage:
   (a) physical—intracranial haemorrhage,
   (b) chemical—hypoxia,
               kernicterus.
2 Infections:
   (a) septicaemia,
   (b) meningitis.
3 Metabolic disorders:
   (a) hypoglycaemia,
   (b) hypocalcaemia.

Fits in the first 48 hours carry the poorest prognosis. Between one third and one half die, and half the survivors have neurological or intellectual handicap. Fits which occur later in the neonatal period are rarely associated with death or serious handicap.

Further reading

Vulliamy D.C. (1975) *The Newborn Child.* J.&A. Churchill, London.
Davies P.A., Robinson R.J., Scopes J.W., Tizard J.P.M. & Wigglesworth J.S. (1972) *Medical Care of Newborn Babies.* Spastics International Medical Publications, London.
Norman A.P. (1971) *Congenital Abnormalities in Infancy.* Blackwell Scientific Publications, Oxford.

Chapter 3

INFANT FEEDING

The feeding of babies has become such a simple business in developed societies that its importance is easily forgotten. Less than 50 years ago in Britain, and today in many parts of the world, thousands of infant lives have been lost as a result of inadequate infant feeding; inadequate in the amount of food provided, in the kind of food, or in the way in which it was administered. The epidemic infantile gastro-enteritis (summer diarrhoea) which used to cause annual slaughter amongst babies was almost wholly attributable to inadequate sterilization of feeds.

Babies treble their birth weight in the first year of life; to treble it again takes ten years. Furthermore, 65% of total post-natal brain growth takes place in the first year of life. Nutrition is therefore more important in infancy than at any other age. Starvation may permanently hamper both physical and mental development. Average nutritional requirements in infancy are:

Water	150 ml/kg/day ($2\frac{1}{2}$ oz/lb/day);
Calories	110 cal/kg/day (50 cal/lb/day);
Vitamin C	15 mg/day;
Vitamin D	400 i.u./day;
Calcium	600 mg/day ⎫ average during first year.
Iron	6 mg/day ⎭

MILK

Milk is a poor source of iron and vitamins but rich in calcium and calories. The main differences in composition between human and cows' milk are shown overleaf.

35

	Human milk (per 100 ml)	Cows' milk (per 100 ml)
Protein	1.2 g	3.3 g
Casein	0.3 g	2.7 g
Soluble proteins	0.9 g	0.6 g
Lactose	7.0 g	4.8 g
Fat	3.7 g	3.7 g
Saturated	48%	58%
Unsaturated	52%	42%
Sodium	15 mg	58 mg
Phosphorus	15 mg	100 mg

It will be noted that in cows' milk the protein content is much higher and most of it is casein: the lactose content is lower: the fat content is similar, but more of it is in the form of saturated fatty acids. The sodium (and potassium) content is higher, leading to a higher osmolality. The phosphorus content is higher. The processing of cows' milk alters the protein so that reconstituted dried or evaporated milks are more easily digested by infants than is fresh cows' milk. Doorstep milk should not be given to infants under 6 months. From 6–12 months of age it may be given, but it must be boiled first if (a) it is not pasturized, (b) home conditions are poor or (c) there is no refrigerator.

Strenuous attempts have been made recently to reformulate infant feeds to approximate more closely to breast milk in regard to protein, lactose, fat, sodium and phosphorus content. The more complex manufacturing processes of these modern milks inevitably raise costs, but it seems likely that the state-subsidized National Dried Milk will be replaced by a more satisfactory product.

For most purposes the fat content is unaltered (full-cream milks) but milks with reduced fat content (half-cream milks) are available for very small or sick infants. These forms should not be confused with full-*strength* and half-*strength* feeds, the latter describing a feed diluted with an equal quantity of water.

BREAST FEEDING

Successful breast feeding requires the active participation of both parties. The baby needs well-established sucking and swallowing reflexes and a good appetitite. These are normally present in the healthy, full-term infant but may be defective in the sick or pre-term infant. The mother needs a good draught reflex, which may take a little while to develop with a first baby. The stimulus to this reflex initially is contact of the baby with the nipple, but later the baby's hunger cry, or even thinking about the baby, may be sufficient. The response is a secretion by the posterior pituitary of oxytocin which causes contraction of the myo-epithelial cells around the alveoli of the breast, with ejection of milk down the ducts to the ampulla. In the puerperium, the oxytocin secreted will also cause uterine contraction, and mid-wives used traditionally to put the newborn baby straight to the breast to encourage expulsion of the placenta. For the same reason, breast feeding may be associated with abdominal cramps in the first week or two.

Breast-fed babies may be fed by the clock (usually every 4 hours) or on demand. Regular weighing is the only means of knowing whether the milk supply is adequate. Crying does not necessarily mean hunger; sleep does not necessarily mean satiation. All breast-fed babies need vitamin supplements. Breast feeding can be a highly satisfying experience for the mother and ensures close physical contact between mother and infant. There is, however, no evidence to suggest that bottle-fed babies are either nutritionally or emotionally deprived. Infant feeding practices seem to be dictated largely by fashion. Mothers may feel that breast feeding limits their social activities, spoils their clothes or ruins their figures. Rich families in past ages employed wet nurses (e.g. Exodus, 2, vii): today the bottle is more readily available. Nevertheless, there are many good reasons for en-couraging mothers to breast feed, and the encouragement should start no later than the antenatal clinic. Breast-fed babies are less prone to gastroenteritis, infantile eczema, obesity, hypocalcaemic fits and hypernatraemic states. Breast feeding, even for a month, gives an infant an excellent start to life. Nobody wants to see unwilling mothers browbeaten into breast feeding, but there is a happy mean between that and the totally permissive attitude adopted by most doctors and nurses in recent years. Experience has shown repeatedly that mothers will respond to information, advice and encouragement.

BOTTLE FEEDING

Bottle feeding offers opportunities to infect the baby, and the preparation of feeds and sterilization of bottles must therefore be meticulous. Bottles and teats may be sterilized by boiling or by immersion in hypochlorite solution: by either method, attention to detail is crucial. Evaporated milks are sterile, and dried milks pathogen-free, until the tins are opened. Feeds should normally be made up according to the manufacturer's directions and should be given either 4-hourly or on demand. The newborn baby will require feeding round the clock, but within a few weeks will drop the night feed. So long as a night feed is demanded, it must be given. Leaving him to cry is pointless and unkind.

Attention to detail in making up the feed is as essential as detail in sterilizing bottles. The scoop appropriate to the milk powder should be used, it should be filled without compressing the powder (unless otherwise stated) and should be levelled off with a knife. Additional scoops, heaped scoops, packed scoops or additional cereal should be avoided. They add extra calories which encourage obesity, and extra solutes which cause thirst and irritability.

MIXED FEEDING

The age at which foods other than milk are introduced is also determined to some extent by fashion. Breast milk is a poor source of iron and vitamins: proprietary infant milks are all fortified with vitamin D, and most with vitamin C and iron. Breast-fed and low birth-weight babies should be given supplements of vitamins C and D until their diets contain adequate amounts and a case can be made for giving a daily vitamin D supplement to all children under the age of 2. A full-term baby will not develop any nutritional deficiency within 4 months of birth, and this is the earliest age at which mixed feeding should start. It is, however, common practice to start earlier—at 6 or 8 weeks—and some misguided enthusiasts start even earlier. The main principles of mixed feeding are:

1 Ensure an adequate introduction of foods containing protein and iron; avoid *excess* carbohydrate (e.g. cereals).

2 Introduce one new food at a time, starting with very small

quantities and increasing gradually if the food is accepted and tolerated.

3   If a new food is not accepted by the infant, try something else. Later feeding difficulties may stem from misguided insistence on an infant taking food that he does not enjoy.

As the semi-solid component of the diet is increased, the number and volume of milk feeds should be decreased. The duration of breast feeding rarely exceeds 3 months in western societies, but averages 2 years or more in developing countries. The average one-year-old will be having three main meals a day, with a small drink or snack mid-morning, mid-afternoon and at bedtime.

FEEDING PROBLEMS

Difficulties with feeding are common. In very young infants they may be to do with bottles, but at all ages they are more likely to do with battles. Feeding mismanagement in early life may present with vomiting, disturbed bowel habit, unsatisfactory weight gain or crying. Most difficulties arise from one or more of three faults.

1   The *quantity* of food is wrong. Both underfeeding and over-feeding may lead to vomiting and crying. In the first, weight gain is consistently poor. An overfed baby gains weight exces-sively to begin with, but may later lose. Overfeeding is particularly common in bottle fed babies, partly because they are often fed to the limit of their capacity, partly because food has a sedative effect, and partly because of the mistaken belief that the biggest babies are the best.

2   The *kind* of food is wrong. The passion for early mixed feeding may lead to small infants being given quite unsuitable foods. Vomiting, diarrhoea and crying will result. A return to a milk diet will allow recovery, followed by a more cautious weaning programme. Changing from one milk to another rarely achieves anything.

3   The feeding *technique* is wrong. This is a common cause of difficulties and can only be recognized by watching the baby feeding. The baby may not be held comfortably; the bottle may be held at the wrong angle; the hole in the teat may be too small or too big; the milk may have been wrongly prepared. Instruction and advice provide the remedy.

One particular form of crying in early infancy deserves special mention. *Three-months colic*, or evening colic, is a very common problem arising in early life and lasting, as a rule, not beyond the age of 3 months. An otherwise placid baby devotes one part of the day, most commonly between the 6 p.m. and 10 p.m. feeds, to incessant crying. He may or may not stop when picked up, but certainly cries again if put down. Attention to feeds, warmth, wet nappies, etc. are unavailing. Theories abound but the cause is unknown. Many such infants derive relief from dicyclomine syrup, 5 ml, at the appropriate time of day.

Dr Benjamin Spock, whose writings have probably had more influence on child rearing than any since Dr Truby King, suggests that at any feed an infant needs to achieve a certain amount of food and a certain amount of sucking. Babies vary in their need for sucking time. Most babies take a feed in 20–30 minutes, but some drain their bottle in 5–10 minutes and may then have filled their stomachs without satisfying their need to suck. Such an infant may solve his own problems by discovering how to suck his thumb. The widespread use of comforters (dummies) in the face of sometimes vehement opposition from the medical and nursing professions suggests that mothers have known this for a long time. Since comforters will continue to be used, just as fireworks will continue to be made and sold, it may be more constructive to stop trying to abolish them and instead try to ensure that they are used safely. Their only hazard is as a vehicle for infection: they do not make teeth protrude. By contrast, the devices consisting of a teat attached to a small reservoir designed to hold sweet, acid fluids have been shown conclusively to dissolve away incisor teeth with startling efficiency and should be condemned outright.

Feeding difficulties after 6 months may result from allowing unsuitable foods, but with increasing age they more commonly result from attempts to insist on the child eating foods which he dislikes. There is a delicate distinction between encouraging the conservative child to try something new, and coercing the reluctant child to eat 'what is good for him'. The mother who sits by the high chair supplying endless diversions whilst she subtly spoons in 'one for Sarah, one for Teddy', is more likely to be storing up trouble than solving a problem. The management of such problems lies in the patient, repeated but firm explanation that no normal child with access to food will starve; that children of some ages are dominated by the need for food, but at other ages it may be a low priority; that wise parents do not start battles with their children that they are bound to lose; and that a mother will often achieve most by doing least.

Some groups of children present inherent problems with feeding. Pre-term babies make no demands and must be fed by the clock. Some mentally retarded children are also abnormally placid and cannot be demand fed: they may also have sucking and swallowing difficulties. Physically handicapped children, especially those with cerebral palsy, may be very difficult to feed because of muscular weakness and incoordination.

Further reading

MacKeith R. & Wood C. (1971) *Infant Feeding and Feeding Difficulties*. J. & A. Churchill, London.

Chapter 4

GROWTH AND DEVELOPMENT

The characteristics of children which most clearly distinguish them from adults are that they are growing and developing. Adults are not growing, except perhaps in girth, and most of them are degenerating. The processes of growth and development start from conception and are influenced by a wide variety of genetic and environmental variables. Growth may be affected by disease: it may also affect the manifestations of disease. For example, if the aqueduct of Sylvius is blocked in an infant, the head will enlarge (hydrocephalus) but the intracranial pressure may not rise very much. If the same event occurs in an older child, the head will not enlarge but the intracranial pressure will rise rapidly.

PHYSICAL GROWTH

Growth is traditionally estimated by weight and height (length in babies) and this is sufficient for most purposes. In clinical medicine other measurements, including the ratio of upper and lower segments of the body (measured above and below the symphysis pubis) (Fig. 8), span, skinfold thicknesses, and skeletal age by X-ray (Appendix 5), may be needed to elucidate particular problems. Growth and development are not necessarily smooth, continuous processes. Weight and height increase relatively rapidly in the early months of life and just before puberty, but at a very constant rate between. The circumference of the head does half its total growing in the first year of life. Sexual development is concentrated into two episodes, at the sixth week of embryonic life and at puberty.

When interpreting measurements of growth and development

it is important to distinguish between normal and average. It is useful to know the average weight of a one-year-old, the average age at which a child walks unaided, and the average head circumference of a newborn baby. It is also vital to know how far removed from average a measurement can be and yet remain within the range of normal. For each parameter there is a distribution curve, and this can be indicated on standard record charts by showing percentiles (centiles) or standard deviations as well as averages (Fig. 9). The 3rd and 97th percen-

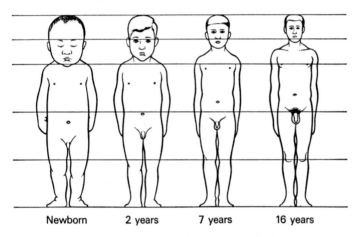

Newborn   2 years   7 years   16 years

Fig. 8.   Body proportions from birth to adulthood.

tiles approximate to ± 2 standard deviations. About 3% of normal children will be below the 3rd percentile and another 3% above the 97th percentile. In normally proportioned children, whether large, average or small for their age, the height and weight will occupy similar positions on percentile charts. Much more can be learned from serial observations of height, weight or head circumference than from a single measurement. The normal ranges for these are given in Appendixes 1, 2 and 3.

The potential for physical growth after birth is determined largely by genetic factors. The extent to which this potential is achieved may be influenced by nutrition, by disease or handicap,

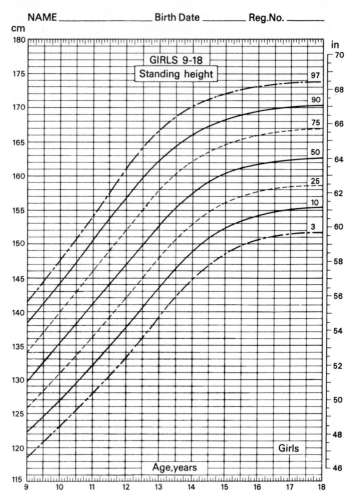

Fig. 9. A growth record (percentile chart) for height. The records contain a similar chart for weight, and are available to cover the age ranges 0–3, 2–10, and 9–18 years for each sex.

and probably also by emotional factors. Failure of normal physical growth is usually recognized in infants by unsatisfactory weight gain (failure to thrive) and in older children by short stature (dwarfism). Sometimes weight gain is excessive (obesity) and very rarely height may increase abnormally rapidly (gigantism).

Failure to thrive

The term is applied to a child in the first year or two of life whose predominant symptom is unsatisfactory weight gain. The main causes are:

1 Inadequate food intake
  (a) Feeding mismanagement or neglect,
  (b) Poor appetite,
  (c) Mechanical problems, e.g. cleft palate, cerebral palsy.
2 Vomiting
  (a) Pyloric stenosis, hiatus hernia,
  (b) Feeding mismanagement.
3 Defects of digestion or absorption
  (a) Cystic fibrosis,
  (b) Coeliac disease,
  (c) Chronic infective diarrhoea.
4 Failure of utilization
  (a) Chronic infections (especially urinary),
  (b) Heart failure,
  (c) Metabolic disorders.
5 Emotional deprivation

Short stature

The majority of children for whom medical advice is sought because of short stature are normal, short children. Some of them were born light-for-dates and many have short relatives including one or both parents. Their rate of growth is normal, as shown by serial measurements plotted on a percentile chart. Most of these children have delayed skeletal development, their pubertal growth spurt is often late and they continue growing for longer than the average. If serial observations of height show an abnormally slow rate of increase, some other explanation must be sought. The main causes of pathological short stature are:

1　Defects of nutrition, digestion or absorption (see page 152).
2　Chronic infections and metabolic disorders.
3　Disorders of bone growth (e.g. achondroplasia).
4　Deficiency of thyroid or growth hormone.
5　Protracted steroid therapy.
6　Most malformation syndromes.
7　Social and emotional deprivation.

Thyroid deficiency in infancy is likely to be recognized from other symptoms and signs before short stature becomes apparent (page 211). Growth hormone deficiency may be part of a wider pituitary insufficiency, the cause of which may be a pituitary tumour, histiocytosis X or unknown, or there may be isolated deficiency of growth hormone. The ratio of the upper body segment to the lower is normal for the age in hypopituitarism: in hypothyroidism the proportions tend to remain infantile. Skeletal development is retarded in both conditions but especially in hypothyroidism.

Excessive stature

Excessive stature is only rarely due to disturbed pituitary function. Usually it is due to genetic factors, the tall child having tall relatives. The prediction of ultimate height is fraught with difficulty, but if it seems likely that it will exceed acceptable limits the epiphyses at the knee may be fused. Hormone therapy is of doubtful benefit.

Chromosome anomalies often affect stature, children with Down's and Turner's syndromes being short and some with Klinefelter's syndrome tall.

Obesity

Obesity in childhood is an increasingly common and troublesome problem—troublesome to the child, the family and the doctor. Some heavyweight newborns seem to have insatiable appetites, their price for peace is food, and they seem doomed to obesity from the womb (Fig. 10). In others, the tendency to excessive weight gain may appear in infancy, toddlerhood or during school years. Fat children often come from fat families but by no means always. Many fat children are undoubtedly gluttons, tucking away excessive calories, predominantly from carbohydrates. Equally certainly, some fat children do not eat excessively but have an abnormal tendency to lay down excess fat. Similarly, some fat children take a lot of exercise, others none. Obese children are nearly always tall for their age. Obesity combined with short stature suggests a possible endocrine cause.

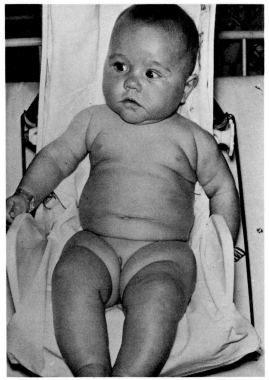

Fig. 10. An obese 4-month-old baby weighing 10 kg.

Obesity may limit exercise tolerance; associated knock knee may lead to complaints of leg pains; and in boys the disappearance of the penis into a pad of suprapubic fat may lead to a mistaken diagnosis of hypogonadism. The dominant symptoms, however, are psychological. The fat child may be teased and ostracized, and the fat girl cannot buy fashionable clothes. There is good evidence that fat children tend to become fat adults, and weight reduction is advisable. The patients and their families

47

are often ambivalent about dieting: they would like to lose weight, but not with sufficient zeal to endure the inconvenience.

For most children, a 1000 calorie diet, encouragement to exercise, and ample moral support form the basis of treatment. Drugs are best avoided; amphetamines should not be prescribed. Any emotional stresses at home or at school should if possible be alleviated. If satisfactory weight loss is achieved, follow-up should not be too short. If necessary, admission to hospital allows the strict supervision of a more restricted diet and weight is rapidly lost. Sadly, it is often regained rapidly after returning home. Finally, obesity is almost never due to endocrine disease and parents need to be told that the child's 'glands are all right'.

DEFECTIVE NUTRITION

Nutritional deficiency may consist in a general shortage of food or in lack of specific dietary factors. Overall food deficiency is only seen in Britain in children who have been grossly neglected, but in many parts of the world, especially the tropics and sub-tropics, *infantile marasmus* is all too common. In these areas, breast-feeding is customarily continued for about 2 years, and there is very little alternative. If the supply of breast milk is inadequate, starvation ensues. The infant with marasmus is a prey to intercurrent infection, and mortality is high. There is also evidence that starvation in the first year of life, even if subsequently corrected, may cause permanent mental handicap.

Kwashiorkor, or protein-calorie malnutrition, is seen in the same parts of the world as marasmus but in older children, usually 2–4 years old. At this age the next baby often displaces the older sibling from the breast, and in many places it is customary to send the older child away to stay with relatives after the new baby has arrived. Food deprivation may therefore coincide with emotional disturbance, and the characteristic picture of kwashiorkor develops. The child is listless, the face, limbs and abdomen swell, the hair is sparse and dry, and there are areas of hyperpigmentation ('black enamel paint') especially on the legs. Diarrhoea is sometimes a feature.

Rickets

Rickets may result from nutritional deficiency of vitamin D or from inadequate exposure to sunlight, or a combination of the two. Rickets may complicate malabsorption states and certain rare forms of renal disease. Normal bone formation requires a proper balance of calcium and phosphorus in the tissues, especially at the epiphyses where active growth is most rapid. Vitamin D is involved in the absorption of calcium from the gut and in the deposition of normal bone. Deficiency of calcium, phosphorus or vitamin D interferes with bone maturation beyond the stage of provisional calcification which therefore tends to accumulate as osteoid tissue. This accounts for the thickening of epiphyses seen particularly at the wrists, ankles and costo-chondral junctions

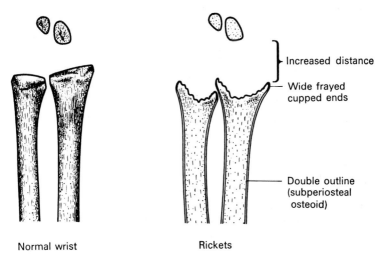

Increased distance

Wide frayed cupped ends

Double outline (subperiosteal osteoid)

Normal wrist   Rickets

Fig. 11. X-ray features of rickets.

('rickety rosary'). The frontal bones may also be thickened, and the long bones of the legs become bowed. There is hypotonia.

In nutritional rickets the serum calcium is normal or reduced and the alkaline phosphatase is raised. X-rays show broadening, cupping and rarefaction of the bone ends (Fig. 11). In malabsorption states rickets is liable to develop after treatment has been started because it is a disease of growing bones. Vitamin D supplements should therefore be given.

Rickets may complicate renal disease under two quite different

49

circumstances both of which are rare. *Glomerular* renal rickets may complicate chronic renal failure mainly because of the failure of the normal conversion in the kidney of 25-hydroxycholecalciferol to the active 1,25-dihydroxycholecalciferol. *Tubular* renal rickets results from a failure of normal tubular reabsorption of phosphate and may be a feature of many inborn errors of tubular function including vitamin-D resistant rickets and cystinosis.

The prevention of nutritional rickets can be assured by a daily vitamin D intake of 400 i.u. throughout infancy and early childhood. Breast milk and fresh cow's milk contain little vitamin D but all baby milk foods and most cereals have vitamin D added. Artificially fed infants are therefore likely to obtain sufficient from their diet, but breast fed and pre-term babies should be given drops of vitamin concentrate for 6 months. Cod liver oil, although traditional, is probably the most unpleasant way to administer vitamin D and is no longer issued as a welfare food in Britain. The liability of Asian immigrant children to develop rickets is due more to nutritional deficiencies than to excess phytic acid. The treatment of established cases requires the education of the mother regarding the diet, and supplementary vitamin D, 5000 i.u. daily, until X-rays show healing. Excessive doses are dangerous. Renal rickets is more difficult to treat and requires careful and continuous metabolic control.

Scurvy

Scurvy is now a very rare disease amongst children in Britain. It is also rare in countries where malnutrition is prevalent because fruit is usually plentiful. In infancy the recommended vitamin C intake is 15 mg daily, although scurvy will probably not develop on half this amount. The predominant symptom of scurvy is haemorrhage, which may occur into the gums, the skin or subperiosteally. The last will cause severe limb pain so that the child does not move the leg ('pseudo-paralysis') and screams at the approach of anyone who might touch it. X-rays show changes at the bone ends readily distinguished from those of rickets, with periosteal elevation and, later, calcification of subperiosteal haemorrhages. There is a rapid response to vitamin C.

SEXUAL DEVELOPMENT

Human sexual development is concentrated into two relatively brief periods of time. Primary sexual differentiation takes place from the 6th week of embryonic life. The gonad, which is undifferentiated up to this time, develops into a testicle in the

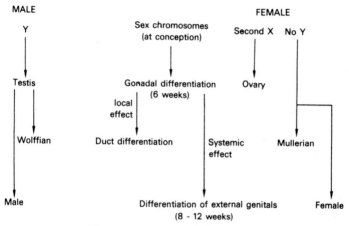

Fig. 12. Normal sex differentiation.

presence of a Y chromosome or into an ovary in the presence of two X chromosomes. The gonad then produces fetal hormones which influence the development of the Wolffian and Mullerian systems (gonaducts) along appropriate lines. The external genitalia develop a female pattern unless there are fetal androgens to masculinize them (Fig. 12).

Secondary sex characteristics develop at puberty in response to pituitary gonadotrophins. The trigger which releases these hormones is still unknown. The age of onset of puberty is very variable, being influenced by racial, hereditary and nutritional factors. In Britain today the age of menarche in girls averages 13 years but ranges from 9 to 17 years: boys mature a little later. In both sexes, puberty is accompanied by an impressive growth spurt. Breast development in girls and growth of the testes and penis in boys, are usually the first signs of puberty. Gonadal hormones are chiefly responsible for these changes, but adrenal androgens play a part (Fig. 13). The progress of puberty may be recorded in relation to the stages of pubic hair and breast development described by Tanner (Figs. 14a and b). Epiphyseal fusion, with cessation of growth, marks the end of puberty.

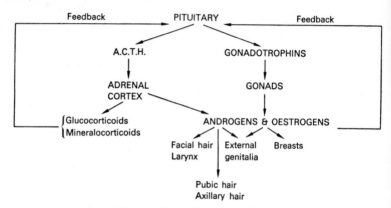

Fig. 13. Endocrine control of sex.

Sex chromosome anomalies

These usually result from non-disjunction of sex chromosomes during gametogenesis in one or other parent. They disturb the development of the gonad much more than they influence the external genitalia and therefore rarely present before puberty except in the case of Turner's syndrome. Most children with abnormal sex chromosomes have normal external genitalia: most children with abnormal genitals (see Intersex) have normal sex chromosomes.

The features of *Turner's syndrome*, which is usually associated with a single X chromosome, are short stature, webbed neck (pterygium colli), broad chest with wide-spaced nipples and increased carrying angle at the elbows (cubitus valgus) (Fig. 15). In some cases there is coarctation of the aorta. In many cases there is lymphoedema of the legs from birth, and this may be the first diagnostic pointer. Secondary sexual characteristics do not appear. The uterus and vagina may be small, and the gonads are represented by rudimentary streaks in the edge of the broad

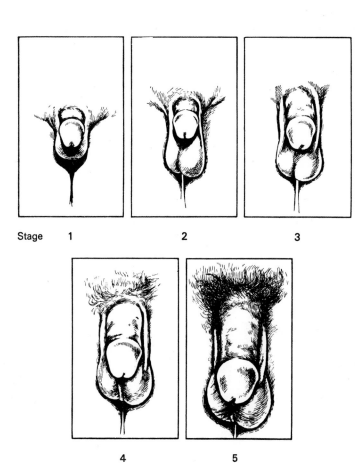

Stage   1   2   3

4   5

Fig. 14a.   Stages of genital development:

1   Pre-adolescent
2   Enlargement of scrotum and testes
3   Lengthening of penis
4   Increase in breadth of penis and development of glans. Testes continues to enlarge. Scrotum darkens.
5   Adult. By this time pubic hair has spread to medial surface of thighs.

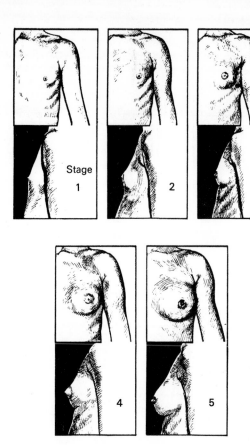

Fig. 14b. Stages of breast development:

1 Pre-adolescent: elevation of papilla only
2 Breast bud stage
3 Further enlargement of breast and areola
4 Projection of areola and papilla above level of breast
5 Mature stage, areola has recessed, papilla projects.

ligament. Breast development and menstrual periods may be induced by hormone therapy, but affected individuals remain infertile and short.

In children suspected of sex chromosome anomalies a buccal smear should first be examined for chromatin bodies (Barr bodies) beneath the nuclear membrane. The number of bodies per cell is usually one less than the number of X chromosomes.

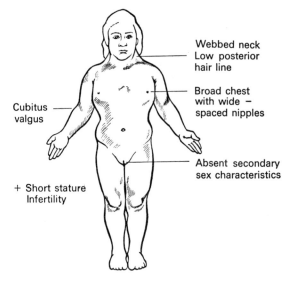

Fig. 15. Turner's syndrome.

The normal female (XX) has one: the normal male (XY) and the patient with Turner's syndrome (XO) have none. If the buccal smear is abnormal, the diagnosis should be confirmed by chromosome studies.

Intersex

The term is used to describe conditions in which the external genitalia are not clearly appropriate to one sex or the other but show features of both. The situation is apparent at birth. Some affected infants are masculinized females; others are incompletely masculinized males. The diagnostic problem is extremely urgent, partly because the most common underlying disorder is a dangerous one—the adrenogenital syndrome (page 214)—and partly because prolonged uncertainty about the true sex is intolerable for the parents: Equally, much harm may be done if the wrong sex is assigned; later reversal may be traumatic. The 'right' sex is determined more by anatomy (functional possibilities) than by genetics.

Apart from the adrenogenital syndrome, causes of intersex are rare. Some progestational drugs given in pregnancy to discourage abortion may masculinize a female fetus. True hermaphrodites (with ovarian *and* testicular tissue) may have indeterminate genitalia. Major pelvic malformations may be associated with abnormal genitals.

Testicular feminization syndrome

In this rare but interesting condition there is a metabolic block in the activation of androgens in the tissues. Affected individuals are genetic males with testicles, but the external genitalia are of a female pattern. Sometimes testes are palpable in the labia majora, or may be found at the time of operation for inguinal hernia. In some patients, normal female secondary sexual characteristics develop at puberty if the testes are left in situ, but orchidectomy is advised later because of a definite risk of malignant change. With the help of plastic surgery these people can function satisfactorily as females, although sterile. It is therefore crucial that they should not know that they are genetically male, or that their gonads are testes. The condition is due to a recessive gene and there is therefore a recurrence risk of 25% amongst siblings.

Precocious puberty

True puberty includes spermatogenesis or oogenesis, and true precocious puberty is rare. Slightly less rare is precocious pseudo-puberty, in which secondary sexual characteristics develop abnormally early, but there is no growth of the gonads and no gametogenesis. The isolated precocious development of breasts (mammarche or thelarche), periods (menarche) or pubic hair (pubarche or adrenarche) is commoner. Precocious puberty occurs more frequently in girls than in boys, and in the majority of instances the cause is unknown. A wide variety of intracranial disturbances, including tumours, hydrocephalus, meningitis and encephalitis, may lead to pubertal changes. Tumours arising in the adrenals or gonads may also cause precocious pseudo-puberty. Boys with the adrenogenital syndrome will develop precocious pseudo-puberty if left untreated. In the McCune-Albright syndrome precocious puberty is associated with tall stature, dark pigmented naevi and polyostotic fibrous dysplasia of bone. Each case requires careful examination and investigation.

THE GENITALIA

Undescended testicles

The testes normally descend into the scrotum about the 36th week of gestation and are therefore usually fully descended in the newborn full-term infant. Spontaneous descent may occur later, but the older the child the less likely is this to happen. If a testis remains undescended until after puberty it will not mature properly and will be sterile. 'Undescended' testicles are often incompletely descended and are palpable in the inguinal canal. If such a testis cannot be persuaded into the scrotum, or if the testis cannot be felt at all, orchidopexy is advised at about the age of 6 years.

Incompletely descended testes need to be distinguished from retractile testes and ectopic testes. Retractile testes are very common and normal. An active cremaster muscle will withdraw the testis into the inguinal canal or higher, especially if the genitalia are examined with cold hands. Ectopic testes are rare and may be located in the superficial inguinal pouch, near the femoral ring, or in the perineum.

Hydrocoele

At birth it is quite common to find fluid in the scrotal sac. It almost always clears up without treatment. In older infants and children there may be a tense hydrocoele on one or both sides. It does not cause symptoms but is often associated with inguinal hernia. Surgery is therefore advised.

Circumcision

The foreskin is normally adherent to the glans in the early months of life and sometimes for as long as 3 or 4 years. In infancy, therefore, the foreskin can only be retracted by breaking down the adhesions, a procedure which is unnecessary for the baby and distressing for the parents. A non-retractile prepuce in early life is therefore not an indication for circumcision. If the preputial orifice is small enough to obstruct urine flow (phimosis), circumcision is indicated. Paraphimosis is usually treated by an emergency dorsal slit followed later by circumcision.

Balanitis is very common in baby boys whilst they are still in nappies. It is a contra-indication to circumcision, and requires treating as for nappy rash (page 175), but mothers often request the operation because the foreskin keeps getting sore. If the request is granted, meatal ulcer commonly follows. Another contra-indication to circumcision is hypospadias because the foreskin is used by the surgeon to fashion an anterior urethra. In any event, phimosis cannot occur with hypospadias.

Adherent labia minora

Sometimes firm adhesions develop between opposing surfaces of the labia minora, probably as a consequence of poor personal hygiene. Urine is passed normally, but the appearance may suggest to the untutored eye that there is no vaginal orifice. The labia may be separated with a probe or by repeated application of oestrogen cream.

Vaginal discharge

Soreness and irritation of the vulva in girls is nearly always due to a lack of personal hygiene. Micturition may be painful. A mucoid vaginal discharge, recognized by the mother from staining of the knickers, results from the normal secretion of mucus in rather larger amount than usual. Careful daily washing and drying of the perineum will relieve both conditions.

A purulent vaginal discharge in childhood is less common. Pus should be cultured and also examined for Trichomonas; the possibility of an underlying foreign body should be borne in mind. *Vaginal bleeding* may occur in infants about a week old due to oestrogen withdrawal. Bleeding in older girls is rare and may be due to normal or precocious menarche, foreign body or tumour. Internal examination under anaesthesia may be needed.

The causes of vaginal discharge are summarized below:

White mucoid (leukorrhoea)
(a) in neonate, normal
(b) at puberty, normal

Offensive yellow (vulvovaginitis)
(a) age 2–5, associated with poor hygiene
(b) infection or foreign body

Bloody (vaginal bleeding)
(a) in neonate may be normal result of oestrogen withdrawal
(b) foreign body
(c) tumour
(d) menarche

Further reading

Tanner J.M. (1973) Physical growth and development. Chapter 7, *Textbook of Paediatrics*, edited by Forfar and Arneil. Churchill Livingstone, Edinburgh and London.

Detailed and up-to-date information about the scientific background to growth and development of children, and all the systems, can be found in *Scientific Foundations of Paediatrics*, edited by Davis J.A. and Dobbing, J. (1974). Heinemann, London.

Chapter 5

DEVELOPMENTAL ASSESSMENT

Developmental testing is now a routine part of the examination of any child. There are standards for the age at which normal children achieve particular skills (Appendix 6). Few people can remember all these 'milestones', but everyone needs to learn a few. The skills can be divided into 4 main categories:

1 Posture and Movement;
2 Vision and Manipulation;
3 Hearing and Speech;
4 Social behaviour.

The starting point is to learn these 4 categories and then to learn one or two skills which fit into each category. There are two parts to a developmental assessment: (a) The history from the mother. The mother is likely to be reliable if a little optimistic about her child's present skills but the older the child the less reliable the dates of the early milestones. (b) Playing with the child—in the presence of the mother so as to encourage the child to show certain skills. The following simple tests require equipment that is available in any surgery or clinic, and require no special expertise on the part of the examiner. The ages given are the *average* age at which the skill is seen.

1 Posture and Movement

Sitting—a child sits unsupported for 1 minute at 7 months, and for 10 minutes at 9 months.

Walking—at 6 months a child starts to take weight on his legs, at 9 months he bounces or stamps when supported and at 13 months he takes 10 steps unsupported.

2   Vision and Manipulation

Visual attention. At 8 weeks a baby observes with a convergent gaze a dangling toy or bright object held 6 inches from his face, and moves his head and neck in order to follow it. An apparent squint after 8 weeks is always abnormal. and requires referral to a specialist. The cause may range from a common defect of acuity to more rare and serious conditions such as cataract and retinoblastoma.

From 2 months a baby prefers to watch a face rather than anything else, but more detailed testing is possible with care and special equipment. The Stycar testing kit includes: (a) a series of white balls of different sizes which are rolled across the floor in front of the baby. At 6–9 months a baby will watch a ball as small as $\frac{1}{4}$ inch diameter at a distance of 10 feet, (b) two sets of miniature dolls-house type toys and cutlery. The toddler has one set and points to the item which is the same as that held by the tester 10 feet away, (c) letter matching cards which can be used at 3–6 years, even though the child has not yet learnt letters. The child points to one of the five letters on his card which is the same as a single letter displayed by the tester 10 feet away.

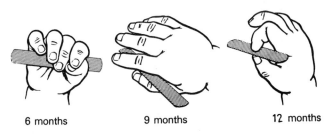

6 months   9 months   12 months

Fig. 16.

Palmar grasp at 6 months,
Scissor grasp at 9 months,
Pincer grasp at 12 months.

Grasp. A wooden tongue depressor or spatula is held before the infant. At 6 months he approaches it with the ulnar border of the hand and then takes it in a clumsy palmar grasp. At 9 months he approaches it with the radial border and takes it in a scissor grasp between the sides of thumb and index finger before transferring it to the other hand and putting it in his mouth. At 12

61

months he approaches it with the index finger and picks it up precisely between the ends of the thumb and index finger in a pincer grasp.

Copying. A child will copy with a pencil the following shapes

	or — at 2 years	□	at 5 years
○	at 3 years	△	at 6 years
+	at 4 years	◇	at 7 years

Building and copying with blocks. Small wooden 1 inch cubes are best. The child will copy:

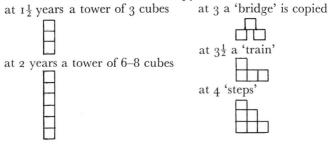

at 1½ years a tower of 3 cubes

at 2 years a tower of 6–8 cubes

at 3 a 'bridge' is copied

at 3½ a 'train'

at 4 'steps'

3 Hearing and Speech

Localization of sounds. The baby is sat on mother's knee facing forward. A variety of soft sounds are made lateral to either ear and out of the line of vision. Rustling soft tissue or toilet paper provides a high frequency sound; a spoon gently scraped round a cup, or a spin rattle are other suitable sounds. At 6 months the baby turns to sounds 1½ feet from either ear. At 9 months he turns promptly to sounds 3 feet away, even if they are situated diagonally (Fig. 17), and at 12 months localizes sounds made vertically above his head. The optimal age at which to test an infant's hearing is 9 months, before insatiable curiosity for new sounds gives way to the contemptuous boredom with which a sophisticated 15 month old treats the tests.

Speech. At 9 months there is varied and tuneful babbling. From 1 year single word *labels* are used for familiar objects and people—'Mum', 'Dog'. At 2 years words are joined to convey *ideas*—'Dadad gone', and at 3 sentences are used. Throughout this period the child's understanding of language is far ahead of his ability to utter it.

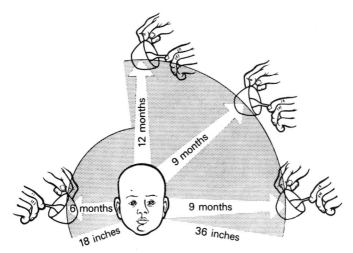

Fig. 17. Hearing responses in first year. At six months the sound should be made 18 in. lateral to the ear. From 9 months the sound can be made 36 in. lateral to the ear (see text).

4   Social behaviour

Smiling. In response to mother's face smiling is seen at 4–8 weeks.

Reacting to strangers. Up to 9 months most babies will be happily handled by anyone, from 9 months they begin to cry or fret if handled by a stranger.

Feeding. At 9 months lumpy food is properly chewed. At 18 months the child cooperates with feeding, and drinks from an ordinary cup using 2 hands. At 3 years he can feed himself efficiently with a spoon and fork.

LIMITATIONS OF DEVELOPMENTAL ASSESSMENT

Technique

As with any examination the expert will always get the most reliable information, but anyone who is willing to listen to the mother and observe the child can get some reliable information about each of the 4 main fields of development. If the mother's account differs greatly from what is observed, it may be that the child is having an 'off day', in which case observing on another occasion will be more reliable.

Range of normal

The age at which a normal child achieves a particular physical or developmental goal is extremely variable. 50% of children can walk 10 steps unaided at 13 months, but a few can do this at 8 months, and others not until 18 months. It is common for one field of activity to appear delayed in a normal child but much less common for all 4 fields of development to be delayed if the child is normal.

Milestones are stepping stones

Parents tend to think of certain developmental skills as essential milestones. It is truer to regard them as stepping stones. In general one cannot reach a particular stepping stone without using the previous ones—and a child does not run until he can walk or walk until he can stand. But different people may use different stepping stones, and occasionally miss one out. Most children crawl before they stand, but some shuffle on their bottoms, never crawl, yet stand and walk normally in the end.

Using stepping stones we may go in sudden bounds rather than at an even rate—children often develop that way, appearing static for a few weeks then suddenly mastering a new skill. If the next stepping stone is a particularly hard one all the child's energy may appear to be devoted to just one of the 4 fields of development, whilst the other 3 seem static; posture and movement skills may advance rapidly about the age of 1 year as walking is mastered, whilst hearing and speech development appear static.

The first six months

This is the most difficult time to assess the baby, because it is not until about 6 months that many of the easier developmental tests can be used. Therefore, developmental testing before the age of six months is less reliable than at any other time.

THE SLOW CHILD

'He is slow at walking', 'She is late at talking'. Such worries are common reasons for parents consulting the doctor. Usually the parents are correct that their child is later than average at achieving a particular skill. The cause will be found in one of the following 6 categories.

1   motor fault;
2   sensory fault;
3   learning fault (low intelligence);
4   psychological fault;
5   social deprivation;
6   late normal.

In general practice the commonest reason is 'late normal', that is a normal child who happens to be at one end of the age range at which that skill is achieved. But one cannot reassure the parents that the reason is 'late normal' until a history and examination have excluded the other reasons. For instance if the child of 2 does not say words is it:

1   motor—is he unable to use the palate and larynx because of cerebral palsy?
2   sensory—is he deaf?
3   learning—is he of low intelligence, i.e. mentally handicapped?
4   psychological—is there severe psychological illnesses (autism may present as slowness in talking)?
5   social—has the child been exposed to speech, or been left all day in the care of a baby minder who speaks a different language from the parents?
6   late normal?

Speech disorders

Medical advice may be sought about children who do not talk, or about those who talk but have defective speech. Some children have a sizeable vocabulary before their first birthday, while others say little until 3 or 4 years of age. If talking is delayed it is important to search for a reason as described above. In most instances there are no specific barriers to speech and it will develop naturally. In this case it is important to explain to parents how they can help or hinder. Being spoken and read to and mixing with talkative children will encourage speech development. Coercion ('You can't have it if you don't say it'), will delay it further.

Articulation disorders are common. Substitution of consonants (dyslalia) is particularly common. A few substitutions and omissions are a normal feature of speech development (tweet for sweet, poon for spoon), but extensive and persisting substitutions render the child unintelligible and he becomes frustrated by the apparent stupidity of others. Speech therapy helps.

Stammer is also a normal phase in language development. Some intelligent 2-year-olds have so much to say that the ideas trip over each other on the way out. If the stammer is 'physiological', the less attention that is drawn to it the better. If it is more severe or persistent the speech therapist will guide the parents in management and prevent the stammer becoming permanent.

School difficulties

If a healthy child of normal intelligence and good vision and hearing has educational difficulties, an emotional problem will often be found. There may be unhappiness at home; or at school —from bullying or fear of a teacher. In addition to these common problems there are certain uncommon developmental disorders such as dyslexia. A child with *dyslexia* has great difficulty in recognizing written words, though he has normal vision and intelligence. Such children are frequently left handed or ambidextrous. At school their reading and writing are disproportionately bad, so that they require skilled help to compensate for their serious handicap. A report from the school is an important part of the developmental assessment of the school child.

Further reading

Sheridan, Mary. (1960) *The Developmental Progress of Infants and Young Children.* Her Majesty's Stationery Office, London.

Egan D., Illingworth R.S. & MacKeith R.C. (1965) Developmental Screening 0–5. *Clinics in Developmental Medicine No. 20.* W. Heinemann Medical Books.

Illingworth R.S. (1972) *The Development of the Infant and Young Child.* Livingstone, Edinburgh and London.

Chapter 6

THE NERVOUS SYSTEM

Brain growth occurs early in life, and is largely complete by the age of 2 years. Myelination is mainly complete by the age of 3, but both myelination and arborization (the establishment of dendritic connections) continue to a small extent up to the age of 5.

Conventional examination of the nervous system has to be modified considerably for children, particularly young children. As is the case with so many childhood examinations careful *inspection* is of great importance. A few minutes spent sitting near the young child, observing him closely may yield as much information as the rest of the examination. In the baby, the doctor is observing posture and movement, and looking for abnormal postures, for the level of spontaneous activity, for abnormal movements and asymmetry of movement. The toddler is best watched at play, particular interest being paid to gait and manipulative skills; ataxia, tremors, abnormal hand postures or weakness of a limb are easily seen. Much more information is gleaned from detailed observation of the contented infant or toddler at play, than from the unhappy young child who is thrust supine on a bed and subjected to a conventional adult type of neurological examination, even though certain aspects of such an examination are helpful in children as well as adults.

Assessment of *tone* is particularly useful, and it is worth handling many young children to become familiar with normal tone. A child's tendon *reflexes* are more easy to elicit in the legs than in the arms. The plantar reflex elicited by stimulating the lateral border of the sole is extensor in infants, and does not become flexor until 1–2 years of age.

The fundi may be difficult to see in uncooperative children. Older children will keep their eyes still whilst being examined, but with younger children it is more realistic to aim at them keeping their head fairly still. Young children struggle against having their eyelids held apart, and the doctor is more likely to see the fundi of a 3-year-old if he keeps his hands off the child's face altogether. In contrast firm assisting hands are always needed to examine an infant's fundi, or those of a struggling toddler, and it is frequently necessary both to sedate the infant beforehand and to apply a mydriatic such as tropicamide in order to see the fundi satisfactorily.

The neurological examination of infants has to include some additional items:

The Head

The maximum occipito-frontal *head circumference* is noted and compared with the normal on a percentile chart (Appendix 1). The fontanelles are palpated. The *anterior* fontanelle closes between 12 and 18 months. It should feel soft. A bulging or tense fontanelle is common in crying infants; in a quiet infant it is a sign of raised intracranial pressure.

Primitive reflexes

These reflexes are present in early life but disappear as myelination is completed and cortical control develops. They vary in intensity during the early months, start to go from 3 months and should be gone by 6 months. A strongly positive primitive reflex after 6 months indicates cerebral damage or severe subnormality. Examples of such primitive reflexes are:

(a) The Moro reflex which occurs in response to many stimuli. One method of eliciting it is to hold the baby supine with the head supported in one hand. When the head is allowed to drop 2 inches the arms and legs abduct and extend. The movement should be symmetrical.

(b) The plantar and palmar grasp reflexes, in which flexion of the fingers or toes occurs in response to a finger being pressed on the palm or sole respectively, and is released by pressure along the extensor surface of the fingers or toes.

(c) Asymmetrical tonic neck reflex. As the infant turns his head to the side, the limbs on the chin side extend and those on the occipital side flex. This reflex is maximal at the age of 3 months.

There is sometimes confusion between the neurological

examination of infants and developmental assessment. Both are equally important, but though they are linked with each other it is best to consider and record them separately. Developmental assessment (Chapter 5) is primarily concerned with the achievement of learnt skills. Neurological examination is primarily concerned with normal and abnormal anatomy and physiology of the nervous system. Primitive reflexes, for instance, are involuntary reactions to stimuli (some people call them 'infantile automatisms'), and even though they develop and change during the early months they are best included in the neurological examination rather than the developmental assessment.

CONVULSIONS

The pattern and prognosis of convulsions varies greatly with age.

1   Neonatal period 0–1 month

Convulsions are common, the main causes being birth injury and hypoglycaemia on days 1 and 2 and hypocalcaemia on days 4–8 (further details are given on page 34).

2   Early infancy 1–6 months

Convulsions are rare and of serious prognosis. They are likely to be a sign of a severe cerebral insult such as meningitis or cerebral malformation. *Infantile Spasms* are a particular form of convulsion that start in this age range. The infant doubles up, flexing at the waist and neck, and flinging the arms forward—a 'salaam' spasm; less commonly it is an extensor spasm. Associated mental subnormality is common. The EEG usually shows a characteristically disorganized picture—hypsarrhythmia. Corticosteroids may suppress the fits. The final outcome is related to the cause which may be a metabolic fault, a congenital structural abnormality of the brain or various other forms of brain damage, including encephalopathy after pertussis immunization. Quite often no cause is found.

3   The pre-school child 6 months–5 years

At this age 4% of children have a convulsion. The commonest form is a *Febrile Convulsion*. They are most common between the ages of 6 months and 3 years, and should not be diagnosed over the age of 5. A family history of febrile convulsions or epilepsy is present in 20%.

The convulsion is usually generalized with clonic movements lasting from 1 to 20 minutes; most are brief. They are precipitated by a febrile illness, particularly upper respiratory tract infection, and tend to occur early in the course of the illness. The CSF is normal, and there are no neurological signs once the convulsion has ceased. The EEG is usually normal. Half the children will have repeat febrile convulsions with future illnesses, but less than 20% have convulsions after the age of 5. Prolonged convulsions, frequent convulsions or an abnormal EEG make fits in later life (i.e. epilepsy) more likely.

Immediate therapy consists of:

(a) cooling the child. Antipyretics such as aspirin are helpful. Concerned parents will often have put extra bed clothes on the ill child and ceremonially lit the fire in the back bedroom. The child needs to be removed from this furnace.

(b) antibiotics, if an infection such as otitis media is discovered.

(c) anticonvulsants, which are continued while the child is febrile.

The main problem for the doctor is in deciding whether to admit the child to hospital. If there is any suspicion of meningitis, admission is necessary for lumbar puncture. If there is clear evidence of an associated infection home treatment is reasonable particularly if there is a previous history of febrile convulsions.

4 Schoolchild 5–15 years

'Idiopathic' epilepsy is the usual reason for convulsions at this age. The child is healthy and normal but has recurrent convulsions. The three main categories of epilepsy are:

Grand mal

These are major fits which classically have an aura, tonic phase, clonic phase then sleep. Abbreviated forms of grand mal are common. Occasionally the fit is associated with and followed by transient hemiparesis (Todd's paresis) which resolves within 12 hours. Although most fits are idiopathic it is important to search for a primary cause from a careful history and examination, for fits can be caused by space occupying lesions, meningitis, hypoglycaemia and many other causes. Phenytoin, phenobarbitone, primidone or sodium valproate are commonly used to control fits.

Petit mal

This is a very brief absence of awareness lasting less than 5 seconds accompanied by eye blinking. The child does not fall down. Petit mal can be provoked by encouraging the child to hyperventilate. Petit mal is uncommon and rarely starts in adult life; the characteristic EEG is a 3 per second spike and wave pattern. It is never caused by organic brain damage, and the intelligence and behaviour of the child are normal. Ethosuximide has emerged as the drug of first choice.

Temporal lobe epilepsy (psychomotor epilepsy)

This is common; it may present as motor, sensory, or emotional phenomena singly or in combination. It is a common reason for minor fits, more common than petit mal. The diagnosis is confirmed by EEG. It frequently results from previous cerebral injury. The children often have behaviour problems, and occasionally impaired intelligence. Sulthiame or carbamezapine is used; phenytoin and phenobarbitone are also effective.

General management of epilepsy

The usual policy is to give the lowest dose of anticonvulsant that suppresses fits and to continue the drug until 2 years after the last fit. Compared with adult anticonvulsant therapy one important difference is that phenobarbitone causes hyperkinesis and behaviour problems in many children with epilepsy; for this reason phenytoin may be preferred.

Most children with epilepsy attend normal school; only a tiny minority have such intractable epilepsy that special schooling is required. It is important that the teachers are informed so that they may recognize and deal with any fit. Although the child should take part in most activities he may need extra supervision for swimming, and it may be wisest to prevent him from doing activities such as rope climbing during physical education.

Status epilepticus refers to the state in which a child convulses or has a series of convulsions for over 20 minutes without recovering consciousness in between. Apart from external injury, brain damage may result. Therefore all fits must be stopped fast. Intravenous diazepam is the drug of choice in hospital. At home intramuscular diazepam can be used or intramuscular paraldehyde (using a glass syringe).

Conditions simulating epilepsy

Breath holding attacks (p. 106).

Faints are uncommon below the age of 10, but common in adolescent school girls. In contrast to fits the girl remembers feeling dizzy beforehand, and is not sleepy afterwards. Pallor and sweating may accompany the faint.

Masturbatory episodes in infants and toddlers may mimic fits. The child may sit or lie with legs squeezed together, or rock to and fro. He may be flushed, breathless or may utter a shriek.

Acute infantile hemiplegia presents as a fit, but is a rare and serious condition. A previously healthy young child has severe convulsions, often unilateral, becomes comatose and develops hemiplegia. Vascular causes are suspected but rarely identified. Recovery is slow and incomplete in that the child usually has residual weakness of one side, intellectual impairment or epilepsy.

Night terrors (p. 105).

MENINGITIS

The onset is generally sudden. In infancy there is fever, irritability and vomiting and the older child will complain of head and neck ache in addition. Fits are common and increasing drowsiness precedes coma.

In infancy the main sign of meningitis is a bulging anterior fontanelle; head retraction is common but it is difficult to elicit neck stiffness in infants. Older children do have pronounced neck stiffness and this is best demonstrated by persuading the child to look down at an object, to press the examiners finger against his chest with his chin, or to kiss his own knees. This is a more reliable method than the examiner forcefully flexing the child's head, as many children without meningitis resist this.

Common viral causes of meningitis (aseptic meningitis) are mumps and ECHO viruses. Mumps meningitis often occurs in the absence of other manifestations of mumps and is especially common in boys. Poliomyelitis, once a common and serious form of aseptic meningitis, is hardly ever seen in countries which provide mass immunization against the disease. Bacterial causes of meningitis (purulent meningitis) are slightly less common than viral causes but more serious and more likely to cause brain injury. In the neonate *E. coli* is the commonest cause of meningitis, but thereafter the three main pathogens are the meningococcus, haemophilus influenzae and the pneumococcus.

Investigation

Any child in whom there is any suspicion of meningitis must be admitted immediately to hospital. Prompt lumbar puncture is imperative. Usually it is possible to differentiate an aseptic meningitis from a purulent meningitis from the CSF examination (Table 5).

Table 5. Characteristics of CSF

	Normal	Aseptic Meningitis	Purulent Meningitis
Appearance	Clear	Clear or hazy	Cloudy or purulent
Cells/cmm	0–4	20–1,000	1,000–5,000
Type	Lymphocytes	Lymphocytes	Polymorphs
Protein g/l	0.2–0.4	0.2–1.0	0.4–10
Glucose mmol/l	3–6	3–6	0.5–6

The difference is not always as distinct as shown in the table and when the findings are equivocal it is usual to treat as if there is a bacterial pathogen. Tuberculous meningitis (page 241) may present initially as an aseptic meningitis. Direct microscopic examination of the CSF frequently leads to immediate identication of bacteria (e.g. Gram-negative diplococci are almost

certainly meningococci); in other cases culture leads to identification. Faeces, CSF and throat swabs can be cultured for viruses,
and in all cases blood culture should be performed. The ESR
may be of help in meningitis, for a value of over 50 makes a viral
aetiology (aseptic meningitis) most improbable.

Treatment

Children with purulent meningitis are treated initially with intravenous antibiotics. Until the bacterium has been identified triple
therapy with penicillin, sulphadimidine and chloramphenicol
may be used. This is combined with whatever supportive and
symptomatic therapy may be needed—anticonvulsants, analgesics, or intravenous fluids for a collapsed child. Improvement
should occur within 36 hours, and early treatment is usually
associated with complete recovery. Slow recovery or relapse may
be a sign of a subdural effusion. Aspiration and drainage of the
effusion is then needed.

Outcome

Meningitis is a serious condition. Nearly 10% of children die
and a proportion incur permanent brain damage resulting in
deafness, mental handicap or cerebral palsy. These problems
and secondary hydrocephalus are more likely in infants. Aseptic
meningitis is treated symptomatically and has a lower incidence
of complications. Recurrent meningitis is most rare, and should
provoke a close search for a dermal sinus. These are small pits
found in the midline of the back which provide a portal through
which microorganisms reach the meninges.

Meningococcal septicaemia

This may occur with or without associated meningitis. It is a
serious and frightening condition which is endemic in Britain.
Small epidemics sometimes occur, though the infectivity within
households is low. Pre-school children are most severely affected.
The onset is abrupt and the course may be catastrophically
fulminating with death occurring within 12 hours. The patho-
gnomic sign is a profuse purpuric rash; sometimes the lesions

coalesce to form large ecchymoses. One mode of death is from collapse as a result of haemorrhage into the adrenal glands (Waterhouse–Friederichsen syndrome). An intravenous infusion should be set up on any child suspected of having meningococcal septicaemia; antibiotics are given intravenously, and the line can be used for plasma expanders or hydrocortisone in the event of collapse.

Encephalitis

Encephalitis is an illness in which cerebral symptoms (e.g. fits and drowsiness) or neurological signs are not accompanied by definite signs of meningitis. The CSF usually has raised protein or lymphocytes. The commonest form of encephalitis in childhood is acute disseminated encephalomyelitis associated with infection (also called meningo-encephalitis). It is not caused by direct infective invasion of the brain, and usually occurs about a week after one of the common infectious fevers—measles, rubella, chicken pox or mumps, or after smallpox vaccination. Most cases are mild, but occasionally severe and permanent brain damage results.

Meningism

This is the term given to the symptoms and signs, particularly the neck stiffness, that may be present at the time of an extra-cranial infection. It may be associated with otitis media, tonsillitis, cervical adenitis or pneumonia. Often a lumbar puncture has to be done to ensure that the CSF is normal and the child has not got meningitis.

HYDROCEPHALUS

Hydrocephalus arises from obstruction to the normal CSF circulation either as a result of congenital abnormality, e.g. aqueduct stenosis, or from post-natal causes such as meningitis, intracranial haemorrhage or tumour. It is commonly associated with spina bifida.

In congenital hydrocephalus the size of the head at birth varies from normal to such gross enlargement that the infant can only be delivered after destruction of the skull.

As the CSF accumulates under pressure the head enlarges rapidly, the skull sutures separate, the anterior fontanelle bulges and the scalp veins appear prominent. In the older child whose skull sutures are united, obstruction to CSF causes headache, vomiting and other symptoms of raised intracranial pressure. It is the rate of skull expansion rather than any single skull circumference measurement that has to be measured in order to differentiate the infant with hydrocephalus from the normal infant with a big head (Fig. 18).

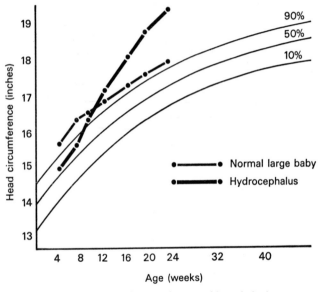

Fig. 18. The head circumference of a normal large baby increases at a rate parallel to the percentile lines; that of the hydrocephalic increases at an abnormal rate.

Untreated hydrocephalus leads to permanent brain injury, therefore surgical treatment should be prompt. The usual practice is to bypass the obstruction by inserting a Spitz-Holter or a Pudenz valve. This is a catheter with a one-way valve, one end of which is inserted into the lateral ventricle whilst the other is passed via the internal jugular vein into the right atrium (Fig. 19) or into the peritoneal cavity. Depending on the cause of the obstruction and the speed of treatment, normal brain development and function is possible. Low grade infection and other technical problems often prevent the valves from being as permanently effective as desired.

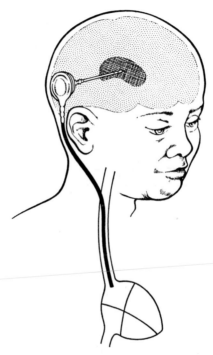

Fig. 19. Pudenz valve draining CSF from the lateral ventricle into the right atrium.

SPINA BIFIDA

This is a common and important congenital defect resulting from failure of closure of the posterior neuropore, which normally occurs around the 27th day of embryonic life. It occurs more commonly amongst whites (Europeans and Americans) than amongst negroes, and is more frequent in families living in poor socio-economic circumstances.

The commonest and most severe form is a *Meningomyelocele* (myelocele) in which elements of the spinal cord and nerve roots are involved. It may occur at any spinal level but the usual site is the lumbar region. The baby is born with a raw swelling over the spine in which malformed spinal cord is either exposed

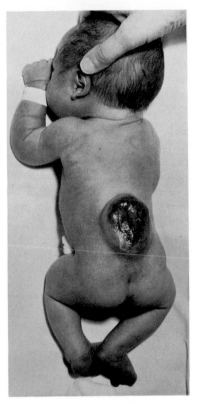

Fig. 20. Meningomyelocele, shortly after birth.

or covered by a fragile membrane. The cord is at risk of further damage from infection, drying out or other direct physical trauma (Fig. 20).

The majority are associated with hydrocephalus, particularly as a result of the Arnold-Chiari malformation in which a tongue of malformed medulla and cerebellum protrudes down through the foramen magnum.

The main physical problems from meningomyelocele are:

1 Legs—partial or complete paralysis below the level of the lesion, with associated sensory loss. Secondary hip dislocation and leg deformities occur.

2 Head—associated hydrocephalus with possible brain damage.

3 Bladder—neurogenic bladder with overflow incontinence and recurrent urinary tract infections leading to kidney damage.

In addition, paralysis of the anus will be present if the relevant spinal cord segments or roots are involved. The emotional and social problems for the child and family are massive, varying from the frequent hospital admissions and attendances to the problems of providing suitable education for a paraplegic deformed child.

The policy of the last decade, in which all children with a meningomyelocele had the defect closed by surgery as early as possible, has been replaced by a more selective policy. However, it is essential that any baby with the lesion is transferred at once to a centre where expert assessment can be performed and surgical closure attempted when appropriate. This will protect the cord from further damage. Subsequently, the child may be helped by neurosurgical treatment of associated hydrocephalus. Orthopaedic procedures may improve function, especially of the hip. Urinary diversion operations may prevent progressive kidney damage, and allow continence, but involve the drainage of urine by an ileostomy. The therapeutic programme is therefore formidable, and the majority are still handicapped at the end.

Meningoceles

These are less common and less serious. The sac of CSF is covered by meninges and skin and contains no neural tissue.

Encephaloceles

Encephaloceles are protrusions through the skull usually in the occipital region. They are uncommon, and if large are likely to be associated with severe brain damage.

Spina bifida occulta

This is of little importance. Although there is failure of fusion of the posterior neural arches of the vertebrae, the membranes and cord do not project through it and are nearly always normal. The site of the cleft may be marked externally by a naevus, or a tuft of hair. There are usually no neurological disturbances. In 10% of children, X-rays show a gap in the neural arch, but many of these have cartilaginous fusion rather than spina bifida occulta.

Prediction of abnormality

A woman who has had one child with spina bifida has a ten times increased chance of another such child. Biochemical tests are being developed to predict the occurrence. Normal amniotic fluid contains a small amount of alpha, fetoprotein derived from the fetus. If the fetus has anencephaly (an absent skull vault and deformed brain), spina bifida and certain other major abnormalities, the amniotic fluid usually contains a great excess of alpha, fetoprotein. Therefore, amniocentesis about the fourth month of pregnancy followed by analysis of the fluid, can be used as a predictive test and possible indication for termination of pregnancy.

CEREBRAL PALSY

Cerebral palsy is a disorder of posture and movement resulting from a non-progressive lesion of the developing brain. In general the term is rarely applied to brain lesions incurred after the age of 2 years. Children with cerebral palsy are sometimes called 'spastics', but not all have spasticity (see below). It occurs approximately once in every 300 live births.

The main *causes* can be classified according to the time they occur.

1 Abnormalities of the intrauterine environment include infections such as rubella and toxoplasmosis, and massive irradiation.

2 Perinatal factors are the commonest cause: birth trauma, anoxia, hypoglycaemia, hyperbilirubinaemia.

3 Illnesses of infancy account for 10% of cerebral palsy: meningitis and encephalitis, trauma and vascular accidents.

Low birth weight is an important associated factor, for one third of all children with cerebral palsy were low birth weight babies.

The *presentation* varies according to the severity. In the most severe cases poor sucking or altered muscle tone may arouse suspicion soon after birth. More often cerebral palsy is first suspected around the age of 6 months when the child's motor

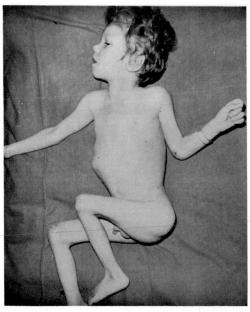

Fig. 21. A three-year-old boy with spastic quadriplegia. His hips are flexed and adducted, and his arms still show the asymmetric tonic neck reflex.

development is delayed—he may have poor head control or be late at sitting. It is important to realize that although the brain lesion is fixed and non-progressive, the disorder it causes varies in the early years as different movement patterns are acquired. Thus an affected infant is often floppy and hypotonic up to the age of 6 months and then becomes hypertonic.

There are 3 main *types of cerebral palsy*

1 Spasticity. Defined as a persistent increase of stretch reflexes

resulting in increased tone which is found only in one direction of joint movement ('Clasp-knife'). Stretch produces a feeling of increased muscular resistance which characteristically may lessen abruptly ('catch and give reaction'). It is still present during sleep. Tendon reflexes are increased and clonus may be present. The spasticity may be sub-classified according to the limbs involved:

Quadriplegia—of 4 limbs (Fig. 21). Other terms also are applied to this state: tetraplegia, diplegia (when the legs are more spastic than the arms) and double hemiplegia (when the arms are worst affected).

Hemiplegia—arm and leg of the same side.

Paraplegia—both legs.

2 Involuntary movements. Choreoathetosis, a mixture of choreic and athetoid movements is commonest. These irrepressible movements are exacerbated by voluntary movement, and are absent during sleep. They are frequently associated with dystonia (disordered posture with varying hypo- and hypertonicity).

3 Ataxia. This unsteadiness of normal movements is often associated with incoordination, intention tremor and poor balance. Cerebellar lesions are a common cause.

Some children have mixed disorders incorporating features from 2 or even 3 of these types of cerebral palsy.

Management

The managment of these children is a difficult art. Early comprehensive assessment is essential, firstly because the factors which cause cerebral palsy may cause other serious defects, e.g. mental handicap or epilepsy, and secondly because disordered movement can lead to secondary problems, e.g. joint deformities or home and educational problems. Therefore apart from a detailed history and general examination the following have to be assessed: vision, hearing and intelligence, and the emotional and social state of the child and home. The fact that the divorce rate of parents with cerebral palsied children is higher than for any other condition is just one expression of the great stress which such children may place on the family. It is a degree of stress that can be considerably reduced by an energetic and compassionate doctor. Whilst early physiotherapy is designed to prevent deformity, orthopaedic surgery can be of great benefit when deformity has occurred.

Prognosis

This depends mainly on the presence or absence of associated handicaps, and in particular on the intelligence of the child. With normal intelligence the problems of even the most severe motor handicap may be overcome. The quality of the management itself affects the prognosis. A severely affected child may require education in a special school where expert physiotherapy, occupational therapy, teaching and other facilities are available.

Children less severely affected manage at normal school, and the least severely affected of all do not always reach the specialist. Their clumsiness, their inability to march in step, or their difficulty in copying shapes may make them an object of derision at school without it being realized that they are suffering from 'minimal brain damage'.

SPACE OCCUPYING LESIONS

These result in raised intracranial pressure as a result of their own size and by interfering with normal CSF drainage. Headache, misery and irritability are common early symptoms and are followed by unsteadiness, vomiting and visual disturbances. Fits may occur.

In infancy the anterior fontanelle is tense and the skull sutures widened. In older children papilloedema is an early sign.

The most important space occupying lesions are:

Neoplasm (page 207);
Cerebral abscess;
Subdural haematoma.

Cerebral abscess

Focal infection in the brain arises from

1 extension of chronic otitis media.
2 congenital cyanotic heart disease.
3 infected emboli from the lungs or elsewhere in the body.

There is a slow invasive stage during which the child is feverish and complains of headache, followed a week or two later by dramatic features of raised intracranial pressure and focal neurological signs. The CSF at first shows a sterile leukocytosis and later a raised protein also. The ESR is always elevated but there is not always a peripheral blood leukocytosis. The commonest pathogens are streptococci or staphylococci, and early antibiotic treatment can lead to complete cure; but once formed and encapsulated the abscess may only subside after neurosurgical drainage.

Subdural haematoma

Bleeding into the subdural space is usually caused by trauma. Subdural haematomata are commonest under the age of 2, in contrast to cerebral abscesses which are uncommon in infancy. Nowadays one of the most important and common causes of subdural haematoma is deliberate violence—the battered baby syndrome (page 249). The symptoms may present acutely or chronically. The latter are more difficult to diagnose for the traumatic episode may be several weeks past, and the infant may have relatively non-specific features of failure to thrive, low grade fever and convulsions. Unless it is drained the haematoma may enlarge as the blood breaks down and more fluid is absorbed into the sac. In this way signs of an expanding space occupying lesion develop and permanent brain damage may occur. Neurosurgery is then urgently required.

CRANIOSYNOSTOSIS (Craniostenosis)

Premature fusion of one or more of the skull sutures results in an unusual shaped head and may compress the brain or cranial nerves. The prognosis depends upon which sutures are affected; premature fusion of the sagittal suture rarely causes problems.

The cause is unknown. Sometimes there is an hereditary factor, and frequently there are associated skeletal abnormalities. The diagnosis is confirmed by skull X-ray. Neurosurgical decompression and separation of prematurely fused sutures is possible if neurological symptoms or signs occur, or if the head is very unsightly.

It should not be confused with plagiocephaly which is a common variation of normal. The infant's head is asymmetrical when viewed from above, one side of the forehead and occiput being displaced forward. The asymmetry becomes less with growth, and does not cause problems.

ACUTE INFECTIOUS POLYNEURITIS

This is an uncommon condition chiefly affecting children aged 2–10. It is characterized by degeneration of the peripheral nerves and nerve roots. The cause is unknown though it tends to occur shortly after various acute infections. There is an ascending paralysis which in the space of a few days progresses to a symmetrical peripheral neuritis with motor loss, sensory loss and absent tendon reflexes. Provided that the child can be nursed through the acute stage complete recovery gradually occurs.

The CSF is either normal or shows a high protein but normal cell count (Guillain-Barré syndrome).

PROGRESSIVE BRAIN DISEASE

This rare occurrence can be caused by a variety of conditions, many of which are genetically determined. It presents with the loss of previously acquired skills. The end result of progressive neurological degeneration is severe wasting and death, usually from a respiratory infection.

The progressive diseases can be grouped into those which mainly affect the grey matter (e.g. the lipidoses such as Tay-Sachs disease) or the white matter (e.g. metachromatic leucodystrophy). Precise diagnosis may be difficult. It is an important aim because a few conditions may be helped by treatment, and for the majority which cannot be improved, an accurate diagnosis allows genetic counselling for the parents.

Further reading

Forfar J. & Arneil G. (1973). Disorders of the central nervous system. Chapter 14, *Textbook of Paediatrics*. Churchill Livingstone, London.

Paine R.S. & Oppe T.E. (1966) Neurological examination of children. *Clinics in Developmental Medicine and Child Neurology*, *No.* 12. Heinemann, London.

Chapter 7

NEURO-MUSCULAR DISORDERS

The two main paediatric problems are myopathies—rare in practice but common in examinations, and floppy infants—common in practice but rare in examinations.

MYOPATHIES

Any disorder of skeletal muscle in which the nervous system is normal can be called a myopathy.

The muscular dystrophies

These are an important group of progressive disorders which are usually familial and present in childhood. They are classified according to their distribution, severity of weakness and inheritance:

1 Duchenne

The pelvic girdle is severely affected, and proximal muscles more than distal. It presents as a waddling gait or difficulty in climbing stairs. There is often marked lumbar lordosis (Fig. 22). Some children develop enlargement of the calves and other muscles ('pseudohypertrophy'). Knee jerks are absent. This is the commonest type of progressive muscular dystrophy and usually has a sex-linked recessive inheritance. Affected boys lose the ability to walk about the age of 10 years and tend to die of pneumonia or myocardial involvement in their late teens. A proportion have intellectual impairment. They have a grossly elevated serum creatine-phosphokinase level which is present from birth. Most female carriers have a moderately raised level.

2 Limb girdle

This starts in either the shoulder or pelvic girdle. The commonest form of inheritance is autosomal recessive. Deterioration is slow.

3 Facio-scapulo-humeral

This is the mildest of the three and a normal life span is possible. Autosomal dominant inheritance is usual.

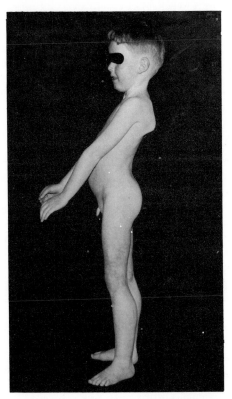

Fig. 22. Duchenne dystrophy. There is pseudo-hypertrophy of the calves, marked lumbar lordosis and winging of the scapula.

There is no specific cure for progressive muscular dystrophy; therapy is supportive but there should be active physiotherapy to prevent contractures and deformity. Because of the many variants and the various forms of inheritance a precise clinical diagnosis is important in order to provide reliable genetic counselling for the immediate family and other relatives. Serum enzyme determinations, electromyography and muscle biopsy together with the clinical picture usually provide an accurate diagnosis.

THE FLOPPY INFANT

Infantile hypotonia is a common problem. Extreme examples are noticed because of paucity of movement; but it is commoner for it to present because of poor head control or the feeling on the part of an experienced mother or nurse that the baby is floppy. It is floppy to handle, and when picked up under the arms the baby tends to slip from one's grasp, and its arms are pushed upwards.

Floppy infants can be divided into two main groups:

1 Paralytic

In the paralytic there is severe weakness accompanied by hypotonia. These infants make few movements and may be unable to raise their arm upwards against gravity.

It may be caused by a number of rare disorders, including spinal muscular atrophy. The most severe variety of this is Werdnig-Hoffmann disease in which progressive degeneration of the anterior horn cells leads to increasing weakness and death in infancy. Autosomal recessive inheritance is usual.

2 Non-paralytic

There is hypotonia but only mild weakness in the non-paralytic. This is the commoner type of floppy infant. In these children it is essential to search carefully for the primary condition causing the hypotonia. The possible causes are numerous:
— Severe mental retardation.

Cerebral palsy—many children who subsequently show spastic diplegia are floppy in early infancy.

Metabolic disorders—coeliac disease, rickets, scurvy, glycogen storage disease.

Certain syndromes—mongolism, Marfan's syndrome, osteogenesis imperfecta.

Benign congenital hypotonia—of unknown cause. The hypotonia is present in the neonate and may be severe. It does not progress, and after a period of several months slow improvement occurs leading to complete recovery.

Floppy infants present a difficult diagnostic problem. If no generalized primary cause is apparent a large number of investigations may be needed including serum creatine phosphokinase, electromyography and muscle biopsy.

Further reading

Moosa A. (1974) Muscular dystrophy in childhood. *Developmental Medicine and Child Neurology*, **16**, 97.

Dubowitz V. (1969) The floppy infant. *Clinics in Developmental Medicine and Child Neurology*, *No*. 31. Heinemann, London.

Chapter 8

MENTAL HANDICAP

Children with mental handicap (mental subnormality) can be divided into two groups.

A   The severely subnormal

They have an intelligence quotient (IQ) of 50 or less, which means that they are unlikely to be able to fend for themselves in later life. They attend schools for the educationally subnormal (severe). Associated physical handicaps and congenital abnormalities are common.

B   The mildly subnormal

They are the majority (85%), and have an IQ of over 50. They can usually manage in classes for the educationally subnormal (normal) and be moderately independent as adults. Although behaviour problems are common, physical and congenital handicaps are uncommon.

Aetiology

The severely retarded are scattered throughout all classes and divisions of society, whilst the mildly retarded are found mainly in families of low intellect and poor social background. It is likely that the poor environment is one of the contributory causes to mild mental handicap.

Mental handicap may be (1) inborn or (2) acquired:
1   The inborn or genetic abnormalities result from
    (a) Chromosome abnormalities, e.g. mongolism.
    (b) Metabolic diseases—usually a single gene defect con-

trolled by autosomal recessive inheritance, e.g. phenyl-ketonuria and galactosaemia. These are rare.

(c) Neurocutaneous syndromes, e.g. tuberose sclerosis (epiloia), and Sturge-Weber syndrome.

(d) Idiopathic—no cause apparent.

2 Acquired. The brain may be damaged:

(a) Prenatally by infection, or more rarely by radiation.

(b) Perinatally by haemorrhage, anoxia, hyperbilirubin-aemia, hypoglycaemia and infection.

(c) Post-natally by trauma, infection and thyroid deficiency.

Presentation

In the absence of gross congential abnormalities the mentally handicapped child is likely to present because of slowness at achieving skills. He will usually be slow in all four main fields of development—posture and movement, vision and manipulation, hearing and speech, and social behaviour (page 60). Sometimes the slowness is marked in everything except posture and move-ment, because of all the skills a baby acquires, those in the field of posture and movement are least related to intelligence. A careful history is needed. It will usually be found that the child has been slow from early life, perhaps smiling only at 3 or more months of age. The child will have been slow at acquiring new skills and also slow at losing certain responses. Primitive reflexes may have persisted beyond the age of 6 months, or the child may have continued to watch and play with his hands after the age of 6 months (at which age normal children have found more interesting things to do).

The rate of learning should be established. Usually the parents recognize that the child is learning, albeit slowly. Specific questions should be asked to make sure that the child is not deteriorating and losing skills. This is extremely rare but very important as it could be a sign of a progressive brain disease (page 85).

Investigations

The history and physical examination may point to a likely cause. In addition a wide range of special investigations may be needed.

These include biochemical investigations of the blood, amino-acid and sugar chromatography of the urine, serological tests for rubella and toxoplasmosis, electroencephalographs and neuro-radiological studies. One of the reasons for trying to identify the cause is to provide genetic counselling for the parents.

Management

Few causes of mental subnormality are amenable to treatment. Usually the brain damage has to be accepted by the family and the doctor, and every effort concentrated on providing optimal circumstances for the child to develop and learn to the limit of his potential. Many of the causes of mental handicap are known to cause other problems. Some, such as intrauterine rubella, may cause deafness and blindness, others, such as anoxia and hyper-bilirubinaemia, may cause cerebral palsy. Therefore any child suspected of having a mental handicap must be comprehensively assessed for associated or secondary handicaps.

Regional assessment centres are at present being established in most areas specifically for handicapped children. Once the problems have been identified plans can be made for dealing with each of them. This is likely to involve many different hospital specialists, as well as educational and social service workers of the local authority.

SYNDROMES ASSOCIATED WITH SEVERE MENTAL HANDICAP

Mongolism (Down's syndrome, Trisomy 21)

This occurs approximately once in every 600 births. The mongol child has 47 chromosomes, because of having an extra chromosome 21. It is usually caused by non-disjunction at the time of germ cell formation, and therefore the occurrence of a second mongol child in a family is uncommon. Less than 5% of mongols result from a translocation fault in the parent; such parents may produce other mongol children. The chance of a woman having a mongol child rises steadily after the age of 35. The father's age is irrelevant.

Mongols are recognized by their appearance. They show a variable number of the following features, none of which is pathognomonic, and any of which may be present in a normal child. It is the accumulation of these features which enables a diagnosis to be made. (Fig. 23).

The skull is round (brachycephalic) rather than egg shaped, both face and occiput are flattened. At birth a 3rd fontanelle may be present just anterior to the posterior fontanelle.

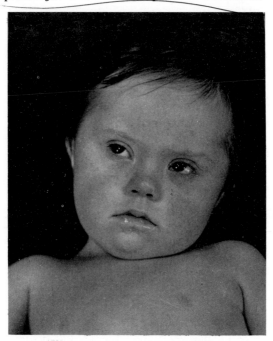

Fig. 23. A one-year-old Mongol.

The eyes have oblique palpebral fissures, with prominent epicanthic folds. Tiny pale spots (Brushfield's spots) appear on the iris in a ring concentric with the pupil. The eyelashes are scanty, and cataracts, squint and nystagmus common.

The mouth is small and drooping. After infancy the tongue becomes furrowed. The pinna may be abnormal.

The neck is short and broad with excess skin posteriorly.

93

The hands are broad and short. A single transverse palmar crease (simian crease) is common as is a short incurved little finger. The feet have a large gap between 1st and 2nd toes with a longitudinal plantar crease running from that gap.

The mongol shows hypotonicity and hyperextensibility. Developmental progress is delayed in all aspects.

Associated congenital abnormalities are common, particularly congenital heart lesions.

Diagnosis

This can usually be made with certainty after examination of the newborn baby. Detailed study of the dermatoglyphics, that is the epidermal ridge patterns of the hands and feet, provides useful confirmatory evidence. Chromosomal analysis is done on the baby if there is uncertainty, and on the parents for genetic counselling.

Progress

Apart from the problem of associated congenital abnormalities, mongol babies may be difficult to feed as infants. Thereafter they tend to thrive, though they have an excess of respiratory tract infections. In general they are severely retarded (IQ 25–50) and cannot expect education more sophisticated than that at a school for the severely subnormal. As adults they will require supervision either within the family or in an institution. Their life expectancy is shorter than that of a normal person; they develop the degenerative conditions of old age (arteriosclerosis and malignancy) a decade or two earlier than normal people. Libido is diminished; no mongol is known to have fathered a child, though mongol females have borne children (half of whom are mongols).

Microcephaly

Primary microcephaly is associated with an inadequately developed brain at birth. The head circumference is small and grows abnormally slowly. The fontanelles close early. The infant has a characteristic appearance: the face is normal but the forehead slopes away so that there is little or no brow to be seen above the face (Fig. 24). Some cases are familial.

Secondary microcephaly is commoner and results from a brain damaged at any time (e.g. intrauterine rubella, cytomegalic inclusion disease and toxoplasmosis, or perinatal trauma).

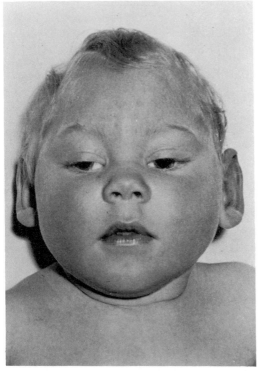

Fig. 24. An 8-month-old infant with primary microcephaly.

Although the skull circumference and growth may be normal at first, from the time of the brain damage the growth decreases and microcephaly develops. The proportions of the face and skull are relatively normal.

Chapter 9

EMOTIONAL AND BEHAVIOUR PROBLEMS

The requirements for normal physical and mental growth have been described in Chapters 3 and 4. This chapter is about the child's emotional growth, the things which may disturb it, and the ways in which this disturbance may show itself. At what age in childhood can one begin to talk about the emotions? Some newborn babies cry a lot, others are placid, but there is no way of knowing whether their different behaviour indicates physical or emotional differences. Sudden loud noises or being dropped may elicit a 'startle' response in newborns, but one cannot tell whether they feel frightened. At 1–2 months the infant begins to become socially responsive, and if a smile is assumed to equate with a pleasurable sensation, one can begin to study emotional reactions.

Probably the most important need for healthy emotional development in the early years of life is constancy. The more widely used term, security, really only means that-which-makes-the-child-feel-secure, and leaves one wondering what it is. A close, personal and physical relationship with one person who provides food, warmth and comfort appears to be the earliest essential. Normally this will be mother, but on occasions it may be father, grandmother, foster-mother, or some other mother substitute. Initially the infant is aware only of mother, but as he grows he absorbs siblings, father and others into his world and begins to establish relationships with them. His horizons expand from mother to family to neighbourhood to school and beyond. At each stage there are new situations to explore, new relationships to establish. Each stage is built on the one before, which explains the crucial importance of the earliest stages.

Constancy implies (a) that a person, and later a group, can be relied upon to provide the necessities of life; (b) that the person or group is constantly available and does not change; (c) that the responses to exploratory activities are constant. It follows that inconstancy arises (a) when the child does not know to whom he should turn; (b) when the composition of the group suddenly changes, or he is suddenly removed from it; and (c) if he receives conflicting responses, for example, in terms of what he may or may not do. In these respects the early months and years are the most crucial time in which the child is putting down his emotional roots. If the ground is constantly being disturbed, the roots cannot grow.

The form which an emotional disturbance takes will depend in part upon the cause and in part upon the child's personality and the family patterns of response to stress. Disorders of eating and sleeping usually result from inconsistent handling by parents. Stress is likely to manifest itself as migraine if the child comes from a headache-prone family. The placid child is unlikely to have temper tantrums but may have recurrent abdominal pain. The toddler who feels challenged by the arrival of a new baby may resort to infantile behaviour.

In summary, the doctor is likely to be faced with two groups of children whose problems are basically emotional. The first comprises those with psychosomatic disorders, in which the emotional stress causes physical symptoms. The second comprises those with overt disorders of behaviour.

STRESS AND ITS SYMPTOMS IN CHILDHOOD

Emotional stresses, in children as in adults, frequently manifest themselves in physical symptoms. These include disease-complexes discussed elsewhere: asthma and eczema (page 178), obesity (page 46), and ulcerative colitis (page 157). Emotional disorder can occasionally be life-threatening, as in anorexia nervosa. Far more common are recurrent abdominal pains, headache, vomiting or limb pains as manifestations of stress. Habit spasms (tics), compulsive drinking and sleep disorders in older children are also usually due to psychological stresses.

The kinds of stress that may precipitate symptoms vary enormously, as does the severity of the stress. Some children are of a buoyant temperament and can ride almost any crisis; others are sensitive plants and bow before every emotional breeze. The following is by no means a comprehensive list but includes some of the stresses most commonly afflicting children.

1 Acute separation. The death of a parent or of a much-loved grandparent, emergency admission to hospital or moving house, are examples of acute separations. These are most upsetting to young children around 2–4 years old who are conscious of the separation but unable to understand the reason.

2 Parental discord. Beyond infancy, all children are conscious of the relationship between their parents and will be aware of any deterioration. When discord develops, the child is likely to be involved and invited to take sides in the contest. This is a devastating experience for all but the most insensitive. A history of recent separation or divorce is not uncommon when children present with stress symptoms, but the symptoms have usually begun long before the break. Indeed, if the marriage is broken beyond repair a physical separation of the parents may provide the only foundation on which to rebuild the child's security.

3 Inconsistent handling. If a child is permitted something by one parent that is denied by the other; or forbidden by parents but encouraged by grandparents; or punished on one occasion and ignored on another, this is likely to encourage the more flamboyant kinds of behaviour disorder such as temper tantrums, breath-holding attacks, and difficulties with eating and sleeping. The intelligent child is quick to play off one adult against another, or to achieve his own ends by alarming or distressing the adults around him. Diplomacy and blackmail can be learned from an early age.

4 Boredom. If children have time on their hands the effect varies with age. The infant who is deprived of companionship and playthings will be delayed in his development. Without encouragement and practice, motor skills, speech and social activities lag. The bored toddler who is confined to his cot 'to keep him out of mischief', having thrown all toys overboard, can choose between cot-rocking, head-banging, pulling out his hair (trichotillomania), masturbating or playing with his excreta. Older children who are bored may take to truancy and vandalism.

5 Sibling rivalry. Toddlers are expected to be jealous of their new baby brothers and sisters. In fact, most toddlers, and

especially first-borns, are absolutely delighted by the arrival of the new baby, but may resent the time which his mother devotes to it. If there is regression or aggression, it is likely to be directed against the mother rather than against the baby. When the new baby is old enough to be mobile and to interfere with the elder sibling's activities jealousy will become more obvious. At school age, constant comparisons between siblings with different capabilities and interests can devastate the less clever or the clumsy. It is almost unbelievable how many parents will discuss their children in their presence, as if they were not there, drawing unfavourable comparisons with other children. This may lead to anti-social behaviour such as lying, stealing, truancy or wanton destruction.

6   Great expectations. Closely allied is the unfavourable comparison between the child's achievements at school and the expectations of his parents or teachers. Parents naturally want their child to do well but may form an unrealistic idea of his capabilities or set their hearts on a career for him which he could never achieve. Although many a child 'could do better if he tried', not every one is destined for an honours degree. If parents constantly nag when he is doing his best, psychological breakdown will follow. Sometimes teachers harass a child beyond his capabilities with the same result. Recurrent abdominal pain, if it leads to school avoidance, may be the presenting symptom, or there may be more serious disturbance, e.g. anorexia nervosa.

7   Acute emotional shock. Sometimes a child is witness to, or involved in, an acutely distressing situation—a road accident, a sudden death, or assault of a young girl. Such an incident may lead to hysterical symptoms (e.g. mutism), to disturbed behaviour (e.g. night terrors), or to acute physical symptoms (e.g. asthma).

PERIODIC SYNDROME

Stress may manifest as recurrent abdominal pains, headaches, limb pains, vomiting or other symptoms. Many descriptive terms have been used—abdominal migraine, bilious attacks, acidosis, cyclical vomiting—and the term 'periodic syndrome' is used to include all recurrent symptoms or symptom-complexes attributable to stress. They are common.

Recurrent abdominal pain is by far the most common of these symptoms, and it has usually persisted for a year or more by the time medical advice is sought. The pain is almost always central abdominal, does not radiate widely, and may be associated with nausea, vomiting or fever. It can be quite severe, the child becoming quiet and pale. It occurs at any time of day, without obvious precipitating cause, but scarcely ever wakes the child at night. The child may complain of pain several times in a week and then not at all for a month or two. As children with recurrent abdominal pain are usually of school age, the parents usually suspect some stress at school. The class teacher, whose report is often helpful, usually suspects some tension at home. Either or both may be right, but often the real reason remains obscure.

Careful clinical examination, including microscopy of the urine, and supported if necessary by IVP or barium meal, must be carried out to exclude organic causes of abdominal pain, and to provide a basis of reassurance for the parents. Constipation can cause pain, usually a pelvic discomfort relieved by defaecation. Rarely, abdominal pain may be the sole symptom of temporal lobe epilepsy. This would be suggested by a history of sleep following the pain, an abnormal EEG, and a good response to anticonvulsants.

Headache is a common stress symptom in children. It is usually frontal, sometimes vertical or occipital. It may be unilateral (migraine) and associated with nausea or vomiting, but a visual aura is much less common in children than in adults with migraine. In most cases, headache is the family stress symptom, and one or both parents will admit to migraine or sick headaches.

Vomiting is intimately connected with the emotions ('I'm sick of it all') but is less common than pain as a stress symptom. It occurs at a younger age than recurrent pains. As young children readily become ketotic and ketosis can cause vomiting, a vicious circle may lead to severe dehydration requiring intravenous fluids and glucose.

After listening to the history, there are two useful supplementary questions. 'What sort of a boy/girl is he/she?' Children with stress symptoms are far more often described as nervous, worriers, perfectionists or solitary than as placid, happy-go-lucky or gregarious. 'Where does this temperament come from?'

usually elicits a rueful smile and the admission that one or both parents are cast in the same die. This helps understanding. Examination reveals no disease, but bitten fingernails may indicate the tension behind the smile.

It is not to be expected that stress symptoms will be spirited away, but much can be given by the exclusion of organic disease (especially the mythical grumbling appendix), by explanation of the nature of the symptoms and by encouragement not to pay *undue* attention to them. It is also wise for the doctor to make clear that he understands that the pains are real and not imaginary. Every effort should be made to identify stresses, and health visitors and teachers can be very helpful here, but often the symptom is being perpetuated by parental anxiety, in which case a careful history and examination coupled with firm reassurance may be all that is needed. Drugs should be avoided.

ENURESIS

Enuresis is a common problem. The term is used to describe inappropriate voiding of urine at an age when control of micturition would be expected. Children learn to be dry by day at about 2 years, and by night at about 3 years. By $3\frac{1}{2}$ years 75% of children are dry by day and night.

Primary enuresis refers to a child who has never been consistently dry. Secondary, or onset, enuresis refers to the situation when a child who has been dry for at least 1 year starts wetting again. Bed wetting (nocturnal enuresis) is a much commoner problem than daytime wetting (diurnal enuresis).

At 5 years 15% of children wet their beds, by 10 years the figure is down to 5% and at 15 years 1%. Nocturnal enuresis is commoner in boys and in lower social classes. Its origins are multiple, and in any child may result from several factors. A genetic predisposition, with a positive family history, is common. Developmental delay may be a factor; just as some children are late walking so some are late at learning to control micturition. Stressful events at the time when the child was learning to get dry may interfere with the learning process and severe stress later in childhood sometimes causes a relapse of enuresis. Most enuretic children do not suffer from either a psychological illness or an organic illness.

Organic causes for bed wetting, such as diabetes mellitus or an ectopic ureter, are very rare. However the child with enuresis should have a full physical examination, if only to reassure the parents who may be convinced that a disease is the cause. If as is usual the child has had a few nights completely dry one can be sure that there is no defect in the mechanics of the urinary tract such as ectopic ureter or neurogenic bladder. The urine should be tested for glucose, and also for infection since urinary tract infection is more common in enuretic children.

Management of the enuretic child is a rewarding art. It is a condition which will go and in most cases an enthusiastic doctor can accelerate the natural cure. Concern and time to listen and explain are vital. Sometimes the home situation with the mother spending the days washing the sheets and the nights changing them is so tense that the general atmosphere of stress and bad temper increases the wetting. Simply explaining to the parents that 1 in 8 of other 5-year-old children also wet the bed will help greatly, and the child will be comforted to learn that at least 3 others in his class wet their beds. Punishment has no place: the children are anxious, indeed over-anxious, to stop wetting. Rewards and encouragement may help. The child can be given a notebook, diary or chart in which to stick coloured stars after a dry night. This chart also helps the doctor assess progress. If the child micturates frequently during the day (has a small functional bladder capacity) the child can be trained to hold on for longer to get the bladder used to a larger urine volume. Drugs may be helpful particularly if the doctor believes in them and makes that belief clear to the parents and child. Imipramine appears to be the most successful. Conditioning therapy by enuresis alarm is increasingly used, and has a high success rate. The alarm is fitted to the child's bed and goes off when the child has wet; within 3 months' use most children either awaken before they wet (and go to the lavatory) or sleep through without wetting.

DISTURBANCE OF BOWEL HABIT

Disturbance of bowel habit in children comprises:
(a) Chronic constipation, which may be complicated by faecal soiling.

(b) Faecal incontinence resulting from neurological disorders (e.g. meningomyelocele).

(c) Recurrent diarrhoea of toddlers, sometimes the result of inappropriate eating habits, but sometimes a 'functional' disorder associated with family stress.

(d) Encopresis: deliberate defaecation in inappropriate places.

Faecal soiling, which is most common at 5–10 years, begins as constipation leading to faecal retention. Sometimes this has been 'deliberate', starting during a negativistic phase of development and precipitated by coercive bowel training. At other times inadequate parental supervision has resulted in infrequent and incomplete bowel actions. The rectum becomes distended with impacted faeces right down to the anal margin. In extreme cases only liquid matter can escape, causing spurious diarrhoea with faecal soiling, of which the child is unaware. His school companions, by contrast, are only too well aware of it, and the child with soiling may become a social outcast.

The abdomen contains hard, faecal masses, often filling the lower half of the abdomen. Rectal examination reveals faeces right down to the anus. There is unlikely to be confusion with Hirschsprung's diseases which usually presents at a much earlier age and in which obstruction is only exceptionally as low as the anus. Unless these is real diagnostic doubt, a barium enema is best avoided.

Management involves first the thorough emptying of accumulated faeces by enemata: suppositories are rarely adequate, and manual removal under anaesthesia is sometimes needed. Bowel training must then be instituted by regular toileting and the use of faecal softening agents such as disodium sulphosuccinate. Laxatives are often needed initially. Instant success is not to be expected because the rectum takes time to resume its normal calibre and sensation. Admission to hospital for 3–4 weeks permits emotional strain to settle down whilst bowel habits are established.

Encopresis is a symptom of serious psychological upset and the advice of a child psychiatrist should be sought.

HABIT SPASMS (TICS)

Repetitive, involuntary movements, involving particularly the head and neck, may occur in response to emotional stress. Tics are not rhythmical and cannot be stopped voluntarily. They are most frequent in boys aged 8–11 years. There has often been a reason for the movement initially—a twist of the neck in a tight collar, a toss of the head when the hair fell over the eyes—but the movement persists when the reason has gone. Entreaties (or threats) to the child to desist only serve to make it worse. Frequent blinking is usually a symptom of stress rather than an indication of any ocular disease. The only possible diagnostic confusion is with chorea, which is now a rare disease. In chorea (page 168) a wider area of the body is involved, the movement is never the same twice running, and a steady hand grip cannot be maintained.

SLEEP DISORDERS

Sleepless children demoralize parents. Young children are demanding by day, but parents survive if they can enjoy peaceful nights. Sleeplessness may begin for a good reason, but persists as a bad habit. Children differ in their personalities from birth. Some seem to be born 'difficult' while others are placid.

Young infants sleep most of the time and crying usually indicates hunger, thirst, cold or pain. It is difficult to be sure of the emotional needs for sound sleep at this age, but the infants of anxious or depressed mothers often seem to be tense and cry readily. A period of wakefulness during the day is common in early infancy (see 3 months colic, page 40).

The most difficult sleep problems are usually seen in toddlers. Some do not settle down when put to bed: others sleep for a few hours and are then full of activity when the rest of the household is sound asleep. By the time advice is sought these habits have usually persisted for a long time and parents have tried both protracted and complicated bed-time routines, and the almost irreversible step of admitting the child to the parental bed. It is always noticeable that whilst the parents often look worn out, the offending child has boundless energy.

This problem can often be traced to one of two sources. It may date from an illness or upset in which a few broken nights were to be expected, but has been protracted by over-solicitous attention. Toddlers are not stupid and soon recognize when they are on to a good thing. The other common cause is putting the child to bed too early or at no fixed time. Children vary enormously in their sleep requirements and sometimes seem to need less than their parents. If put to bed early, either because they are thought to need so many hours sleep or because parents like a little time together in the evening, they are wide awake and resent being confined to a cot.

Sleep problems are best prevented by a sensible routine and a firm line when unreasonable demands are made. Before resorting to drugs it is worth trying simple remedies. If the child is fearful of the dark, a night light or open door to a lit landing may bring calm. If the child demands the presence of mother until asleep, he may accept instead an article of her clothing as a talisman. If bad habits are firmly established temporary use of hypnotics may be unavoidable. Chloral is safe and there are palatable preparations for children. High doses are often needed initially. The right dose (as of any drug) is that which achieves the desired effect.

Nightmares are common at all ages. Parents, having experienced them themselves, are not usually very worried by them. They know that nightmares occur in normal people and that they do not mean major emotional upset. Measures such as leaving the bedroom door open, or a light on, may comfort the child who is frightened of going to bed because of nightmares.

Nightmares occur during rapid eye movement (REM) sleep and are the culmination of a dream adventure, the details of which the child can remember immediately afterwards.

Night Terrors are not common, but are most alarming. They occur mainly in the first hour or two of sleep. The child shrieks, sits up and stares wide-eyed and terrified as if being attacked by something only he can see. He may stumble out of bed and seem oblivious to the parents' soothing words. However, within a few minutes he will be sound asleep again and will remember nothing in the morning. The parents can be reassured that night terrors do not indicate serious psychological abnormality, the child does not remember them, and that the child will outgrow them.

Night terrors occur during non-REM sleep, and occur abruptly (not as the result of a dream sequence). They are accompanied by an alarming rise of the pulse and violent respirations which may at times make the parents or doctor suspect an epileptic fit.

BREATH-HOLDING ATTACKS

Known in Yorkshire as 'the kinks,' and by other names elsewhere, breath-holding attacks are common but harmless. They occur in young children, usually $1\frac{1}{2}$–3 years, and are precipitated by frustration or physical hurt. After one lusty yell the child holds his breath, goes red in the face, and may later become cyanosed and briefly lose consciousness. He then starts breathing again and is soon back to normal. Sometimes cerebral hypoxia is sufficient to cause brief generalized twitching, and the possibility of epilepsy may then be raised. A careful history will usually resolve any doubts. The attacks are benign and self-limiting. The parents require explanation and reassurance. If they can ignore the attacks, this is ideal. If they feel compelled to action, a little cold water over the head (a baptism rather than a deluge) will relieve the tension all round. Sedatives and tranquillizers are not necessary.

SEVERE BEHAVIOUR DISORDERS

Breath-holding attacks, together with temper tantrums, cot-rocking and head-banging, are so common and so benign in the long-term (though causing desperation at the time) that they may almost be considered minor variations of the normal. Severe head banging and rocking may be most marked in children who are sensorily or emotionally deprived (e.g. a blind child in an institution). Disordered behaviour amongst older children and adolescents is often anti-social and therefore much more serious. Such problems are beyond the scope of this book.

Anorexia nervosa

This is uncommon in children, but important. It occurs more commonly in girls than in boys, and rarely before early puberty. In contrast to children who eat poorly because they are depressed, children with anorexia nervosa appear to have an abundance of energy strangely at variance with their microscopic food intake and steadily falling weight. It is a serious disease which can be fatal, and requires hospital treatment under the supervision of a child psychiatrist.

Two contrasting forms of disordered behaviour—autistic and hyperkinetic—merit brief description because they are not uncommon, especially amongst brain-damaged children, and both present important barriers to social and educational progress.

Autistic behaviour

This incorporates certain characteristics of which the most constant are an avoidance of human contact (especially visual contact), delayed and restricted speech and an obsession with sameness—the same things, the same way, the same ritual. Autistic children prefer things to people and avoid your gaze. Sometimes the onset of symptoms is very early: a mother may say, 'As a baby she would never let me cuddle her'. This sort of behaviour is not uncommon amongst children with mental handicap, deafness, or blindness. *Infantile autism* is autistic behaviour in children without other disability. Such children are often difficult to handle and always difficult to teach because of their unwillingness to communicate. An undue proportion of them come from professional homes, and sometimes one or other parent shows mild autistic features—a preference for solitude, an unwillingness to look you in the eye. The condition is so ill-understood that methods of management are still highly experimental.

Hyperkinetic behaviour

In some ways this is a contrast to autistic behaviour. Children vary greatly in the extent of their spontaneous activities and it is impossible to define the limit between physiological and pathological degrees of over-activity. Many normal children are 'always on the go', 'never still', and need relatively few hours of sleep. Beyond this is the hyperkinetic syndrome in which these features reach an unreasonable degree. Hyperkinetic children are bursting with restless energy from dawn to dusk, and often much of the night as well. They move their attention from one thing to another in rapid succession and cannot be persuaded to concentrate on anything for more than a few seconds. They are easily distracted and seem incapable of sustained effort. In children of school age this presents a grave educational problem.

The hyperkinetic syndrome is particularly common in children with evidence of brain damage (mental retardation or epilepsy) which further complicates their education. They need handling with a combination of firmness and infinite patience. Drugs are sometimes helpful. Paradoxically, amphetamine may have a quietening effect while phenobarbitone often makes things worse.

Further reading

Apley J. & MacKeith R.C. (1968) *The Child and his Symptoms*. Blackwell Scientific Publications, Oxford.

Illingworth R.S. (1974) *The Normal Child: Some Problems of the First Five Years.* Livingstone, Edinburgh & London.

Meadow S.R. (1973) The management of nocturnal enuresis. Chapter 21, *Bladder Control and Enuresis*. Heinemann, London.

Chapter 10

THE CARDIOVASCULAR SYSTEM

Heart disease in children differs in many important ways from heart disease in adults. Most of it is congenital in origin, most of it is diagnosed before it has caused ill health, and effective treatment can be offered for much of it. Congenital heart disease is not *a* disease, but a multitude of heart defects arising from many causes. Nevertheless it is a useful term covering all heart disease of prenatal origin. Of every 1000 children born, between 5 and 10 have congenital heart disease. The lesions vary in severity from those which are incompatible with life to those which cause no symptoms and require no treatment.

In comparison, all other kinds of heart disease in childhood are uncommon. Rheumatic heart disease varies in frequency with that of rheumatic fever (acute rheumatism). In countries with well-developed social standards and medical services this disease has become progressively less common, to the extent that rheumatic carditis is now a relative rarity on the children's wards. Primary myocardial disease and subacute bacterial endocarditis are rare. Coronary artery disease and essential hypertension, which account for so much adult heart disease, are practically unheard of in childhood.

EXAMINATION OF THE CARDIOVASCULAR SYSTEM

Although the basic principles of examination of the CVS in children are essentially the same as in adults, there are important differences, especially in infants. The routine examination of the hearts of apparently healthy infants in newborn nurseries and welfare clinics is intended primarily to detect asymptomatic congenital heart disease. The examination of sick infants should include a search for evidence of cardiac failure, which may or may not be due to heart disease.

Cyanosis may be evident at rest or only on exertion, which for the infant means when feeding or crying. In toddlers and older children, minor degrees of arterial desaturation may show as a dark flush on the cheeks, a deceptive appearance suggesting rosy health. Cyanosis due to congenital heart disease is usually associated with clubbing of the fingers and toes, but this is not apparent in the early weeks of life. Breathlessness, like cyanosis, may be evident at rest or only on exertion. It may, of course,

Table 6.   Normal heart rate and blood pressure

Age	Heart rate		Blood pressure	
	Sleeping	Active	Systolic	Diastolic
Fetus	120–160		—	—
Newborn	120	Up to 180	65–110	30–60
6 months	110	150	65–110	40–60
1–2 years	100	130	65–110	40–80
5 years	90	115	85–115	45–85
10–15 years	80	100	90–135	50–90

result from non-cardiac disease, but breathlessness on feeding in a small infant is most commonly due to heart disease. The radial pulses are not always easy to feel in babies, but the brachials and femorals should always be palpable. The sleeping pulse rate can often be conveniently counted by observing the pulsations of the anterior fontanelle. The neck veins are not so easy to study in babies as in adults. Measurement of the blood pressure is important but is often overlooked, partly because it is technically difficult in infants and partly because it is so unusual to find abnormal pressures. In toddlers and older children, blood pressure is measured in the normal way with a sphygmomanometer, using a cuff of appropriate size (about two-thirds the length of the upper arm) and recording the cuff size on the notes. Too small a cuff will give a falsely high reading. Cuffs down to one inch width are available. Alternatively, a reasonable idea of the blood pressure may be obtained by the flush method, which is applicable equally to the arm and the leg. A cuff of suitable size is applied round the forearm or lower leg and attached to the sphygmomanometer. The hand or foot is then exsanguinated as much as possible either by wrapping Paul's tubing round from distal to proximal or by grasping firmly in the examiner's hand. The cuff is pumped up before compression is released, leaving the extremity blanched. The pressure is then slowly reduced whilst a watch is kept on the pale skin, preferably by a second examiner. The point at which the colour suddenly returns to the skin is the flush pressure: this approximates to the mean blood pressure, being lower than the systolic and higher than the diastolic.

The position of the apex beat in children can be referred to the nipple line and is normally up to $\frac{1}{2}$ inch outside it. Overactivity of the right ventricle can be detected by palpation in the intercostal spaces just to the left of the sternum and, in infants particularly, in the epigastrium. Hypertrophy of the right ventricle will cause progressive deformity of the chest in young children, with prominence of the lower part of the sternum and the adjacent parts of the costal cartilages. Thrills should be felt for in the suprasternal notch as well as over the praecordium. On auscultation, splitting of the first sound is not uncommon, and of the second sound invariable if the heart and respiratory rates are not too rapid. Splitting of the second sound is wider during inspiration, and often disappears during expiration. Respiration also affects heart rate, causing sinus arrhythmia. This may be so marked in children that the heart rate in inspiration is twice that in expiration, giving the impression of some bizarre disturbance of heart rhythm. Careful observation of respiration and the effect of breath-holding resolves the mystery. The third heart sound is often easy to hear, especially in older children and adolescents. It may be loud enough to masquerade as a diastolic murmur, but comes hard on the heels of the second sound and is of very brief duration.

In addition to the normal heart sounds, functional murmurs and venous hums are very common in healthy children and are a frequent cause of confusion. The most frequently encountered functional murmur is an early systolic bruit of squeaky quality (sometimes called 'creaking-gate'), loudest at the lower left sternal edge and often quite loud. It varies with posture (examine standing and lying down) and may disappear on deep inspiration. Another common functional murmur, again systolic, is heard in the pulmonary area and is less easily distinguishable from murmurs of organic origin. A venous hum is a low-pitched, continuous bruit best heard beneath the inner ends of one or both calvicles. It can be altered or abolished by changing the position of the neck, and disappears when the child lies down.

A precise anatomical diagnosis can rarely be made on clinical grounds alone except by experts. A good quality chest X-ray and an ECG usually provide additional useful information. If there is any question of surgery being considered, cardiac catheterization and/or angiocardiography are often required to establish the site and severity of obstructions or of abnormal communications.

CARDIAC FAILURE

Cardiac failure is a medical emergency. In children it may result from congenital or rheumatic heart disease; from hypertension secondary to renal or other diseases; from acute or chronic respiratory disease; and from other rarer causes. In infancy, severe respiratory infections (pneumonia, bronchiolitis) readily cause heart failure which may be overlooked because the primary disease will cause tachypnoea, tachycardia, crepitations and perhaps cyanosis. The best clue to heart failure in infancy is enlargement of the liver, which may change in size with remarkable rapidity. There will also be tachypnoea and a disproportionate tachycardia (Fig. 25). Pitting oedema is a very late sign of heart failure in babies. It may be anticipated if daily weighing shows a rapid weight gain in a sick infant. Chest X-ray shows an enlarged heart. The management of cardiac failure includes treatment of the cause (where possible) and the administration of oxygen, digoxin and diuretics. Infants are often restless and require sedation; tube feeding may be needed to avoid the effort of sucking; and skilled nursing is essential. The baby is better nursed semi-recumbent. Dosage of digoxin is crucial as the margin between therapeutic and toxic levels is small, and there is no effective antidote. Initial doses of digoxin and diuretics are often best given parenterally. Infants with congenital heart disease awaiting investigation or surgery often need to be maintained on a daily dose of digoxin for months or years.

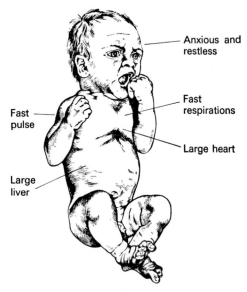

Fig. 25.   Cardiac failure in infancy.

CONGENITAL HEART DISEASE

Circulatory changes at birth

The ductus arteriosus is, of course, a large, functional vessel in all fetuses. Immediately after birth it closes and the lumen is obliterated over the next few days. The other changes in the circulation at birth include the closure of the ductus venosus, and the functional closure of the foramen ovale as a result of the left atrial pressure rising above that of the right (Fig. 26). The precise mechanics of these important circulatory changes have still not been elucidated. The ductus arteriosus is quite often widely patent in babies who have died from any cause within the first days of life.

Aetiology of congenital heart disease

In very few instances of congenital heart disease is the cause known. Amongst the known causes are:

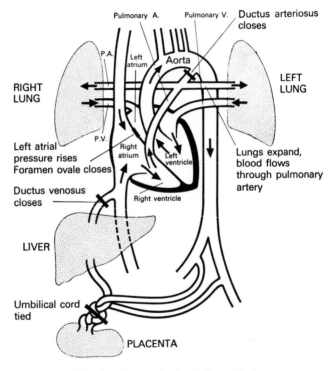

Fig. 26. Changes in circulation at birth.

1 Autosomal trisomy syndromes. Heart lesions are present in about 25% of mongols, and in a high proportion of infants with other autosomal trisomies.

2 Turner's syndrome, in which a minority of patients have coarctation of the aorta or heart lesions.

3 Other rare syndromes (e.g. Marfan's, Klippel-Feil).

4 Congenital rubella. Infection in the second month of pregnancy is likely to affect the heart, and will often affect the eye, ear and brain at the same time. Rubella may cause many different heart lesions, but patent ductus arteriosus is particularly common. The introduction of rubella vaccine should gradually eliminate this cause of heart disease.

In the absence of any hereditary syndrome, the parents of a child with congenital heart disease can normally be reassured about the prospects for any further children they may have.

Congenital heart disease, which may involve the heart, the great vessels, or both, can be understood in terms of disordered embryology. Most lesions arise as a consequence of normal embryological processes becoming either arrested before completion, or deviated from their normal course. The consequence is usually either abnormal communication between the systemic and pulmonary circulations, or obstruction to normal blood flow, or a combination of the two. For example, failure of completion of the interventricular or interatrial septa will result in ventricular or atrial septal defects. Failure of division of the truncus arteriosus in the normal way may result in Fallot's tetralogy, in transposition of the great vessels or in persistent truncus. There may be narrowing of the ventricular outflow tracts, leading to pulmonary or aortic stenosis. The mitral and tricuspid valves are less often involved in congenital lesions, although these two valve rings may remain continuous with one another (persistent atrio-ventricular canal), a lesion which is relatively common in mongols.

Symptoms and signs

The most common symptoms are cyanosis and breathlessness (either at rest or on exertion), difficulty with feeding (which is a form of exertional dyspnoea) and failure to thrive. The most common signs are heart murmurs and evidence of cardiac failure. In general, cyanosis will be present if there is a substantial shunt of blood from the right side of the circulation to the left, but not if there is no shunt or if the shunt is from the left side to the right. Table 7 classifies the principal congenital heart lesions on the basis of the presence and direction of shunt. As the pressure in the left heart and aorta is normally higher than in the right heart and pulmonary artery, an uncomplicated communication between the two sides results in a left-to-right shunt. However, if such a shunt is substantial and is allowed to persist, changes take place in the small pulmonary vessels which lead to pulmonary hypertension and ultimately to a reversal of the shunt. Cyanosis may therefore develop after some years, but should in most cases be prevented by surgical correction of the lesion before the pulmonary vasculature is irreparably damaged.

Table 7. Common Congenital Heart Lesions

No shunt	Left-to-right shunt	Right-to-left shunt
Pulmonary stenosis	Ventricular septal defect	Tetralogy of Fallot
Aortic stenosis	Atrial septal defect	Transposition of the great vessels
Coarctation of the aorta	Patent ductus arteriosus	

Left-to-right shunts

Ventricular septal defect

VSD is the commonest congenital lesion. It may affect the upper, membranous part of the septum, the lower, muscular part, or the septum may be virtually absent. The conducting system is hardly ever affected by these lesions. A high VSD may be associated with other lesions (as in Fallot's tetralogy). An isolated defect in the muscular part of the septum (maladie de Roger) is of special interest because it may undergo spontaneous closure. This is thought to result from muscle hypertrophy, and occurs in at least 20% of cases, usually within 6–9 months of birth. In most instances, a VSD is recognized by the detection of a heart murmur at a routine examination, either shortly after birth or later in infancy. The murmur is pan-systolic, blowing, sometimes very loud, usually maximal down the left sternal border and often accompanied by a thrill. In symptomless infants there are usually no other abnormal signs. A few infants become breathless on feeding from birth or may go into frank cardiac failure. If tided over their early weeks, they may become symptom-free. Chest X-ray may show a little cardiac enlargement, and increased pulmonary blood flow (plaeonaemia).

If spontaneous closure does not occur, operative closure may be needed if the shunt is large and pulmonary pressure high. This is an open heart operation and is difficult to undertake in very young children. Pending surgery, digitalization may be required.

Atrial septal defect

ASD may result from failure of closure of the ostium primum or of the ostium secundum. In either case the flow of blood is from the left atrium to the right, so there is no cyanosis. There is a mid-systolic murmur, usually maximal in the 2nd or 3rd interspace to the left of the sternum, and often not as loud or as long as the murmur of a VSD. The second heart sound shows wide splitting which does not vary with respiration. The chest X-ray shows prominence of the pulmonary arc and increased pulmonary vascularity. The ECG often shows incomplete right bundle branch block.

Atrial septal defects do not close spontaneously and are rarely affected by subacute bacterial endocarditis, but pulmonary hypertension may develop with consequent reversal of the shunt. Ostium secundum defects are high up in the septum and operative closure is relatively simple. Ostium primum defects, in contrast, are close to the mitral and tricuspid valves. The valves may themselves be malformed, and attempts to close the defect usually lead to distortion and malfunction. There is therefore a very different prognosis for the two main types of ASD.

Patent ductus arteriosus

This is the third common lesion characterized by a left-to-right shunt, in this case from the aorta to the pulmonary artery. This is the opposite to the normal blood flow through the fetal ductus. As with septal defects, the lesion is usually diagnosed as a result of a heart murmur being heard at a routine examination in infancy. The murmur is loudest in the pulmonary area, initially systolic but later extending through the second heart sound to become a continuous 'machinery' murmur. This is one of the few murmurs that is absolutely characteristic even to the un-skilled ear, and the only common source of confusion is a venous hum. There is usually an accompanying thrill, although this may not be detectable in early infancy, and a high pulse pressure causing a collapsing pulse and visible arteriolar pulsation. The chest X-ray shows a prominent pulmonary arc and increased pulmonary vascularity; these appearances are similar to those seen with ASD, but the physical signs are quite different.

Patent ductus may cause heart failure, pulmonary hyper-tension, failure to thrive or recurrent chest infections, and may be involved in subacute bacterial endarteritis. Ligation and divi-sion is therefore advised and can be carried out whenever neces-sary. If there is no clinical urgency, it is technically easier when the child is a few years old.

Right-to-left Shunts

The two common congenital heart lesions causing right-to-left shunts and cyanosis ('blue babies') are Fallot's tetralogy and transposition of the great vessels. Both result from abnormal division of the truncus arteriosus. In *transposition*, the septum dividing the truncus has failed to rotate, so that the aorta arises from the right ventricle and the pulmonary artery from the left. This leads to two independent circulations and would be in-compatible with survival after birth. In practice, therefore, there is always at least one communication between the two circu-lations in the form of ASD, VSD or patent ductus, often two, and sometimes all three. These allow some mixture of oxygenated with deoxygenated blood, sufficient to maintain life, albeit somewhat precariously. Cyanosis and breathlessness, especially on feeding, are conspicuous from birth. A systolic murmur develops but may not be audible for a few days. Chest X-ray shows an enlarged heart, often egg-shaped with the apex of the heart forming the apex of the egg and with a narrow pedicle (because the great vessels lie more directly one behind the other than normal). Pulmonary vascularity is increased.

The mortality amongst infants with transposition used to be virtually 100%, and it is still high. Operative correction is now possible in many cases. The prognosis has also been improved by the ingenious and dramatic manoeuvre of balloon septostomy.

If communication between the systemic and pulmonary circulations is very poor, the infant will not survive long enough for surgery even to be considered. It can be improved by the creation of an artificial ASD. A balloon catheter (deflated) is directed through the foramen ovale from the right atrium to the left, the balloon is inflated, and a smart tug on the catheter tears a hole in the atrial septum. The consequent improved oxygenation may ensure the infant's survival for later surgery.

Fallot's tetralogy

Fallot's tetralogy is a single error of development with four consequences. The septum dividing the truncus, instead of joining up with the interventricular septum, deviates to the right. The right ventricular outflow is therefore restricted (pulmonary stenosis or atresia), the aorta extends to the right of the septum (over-riding aorta) and receives blood from both ventricles, and there is a deficiency in the upper part of the membranous septum (VSD). The right ventricle must pump blood either through a narrowed pulmonary orifice or into the aorta (in competition with the left ventricle). It does both, but only by increasing its pumping strength (right ventricular hypertrophy). Cyanosis may not be evident at birth but usually becomes noticeable within a few days or weeks, depending upon the degree of right ventricular outflow obstruction. A systolic murmur develops early, and the pulmonary component of the second sound may be weak or absent. Chest X-ray shows right ventricular hypertrophy and diminished pulmonary vascularity (oligaemia).

Unlike transposition, Fallot's tetralogy is compatible with many years of life, though with restricted exercise tolerance. Older children with this lesion may learn the trick of squatting on their haunches to relieve exertional dyspnoea. Operative correction is normally undertaken in two stages, the first to increase the pulmonary blood flow, and the second, usually before school age, to correct the defects.

Obstructive lesions without shunts

Pulmonary stenosis

This may occur at the level of the valve or of the infundibulum.

There is a systolic murmur and thrill in the pulmonary area, and there may be right ventricular hypertrophy. The chest X-ray often shows prominence of the pulmonary arc due to post-stenotic dilatation of the pulmonary artery. If the pressure gradient across the obstruction (as measured at cardiac catheterization) is only slight, no treatment is needed. If it is more severe, valvotomy or infundibular resection will be required.

Aortic stenosis

More dangerous is aortic stenosis, because it may limit coronary blood flow whilst increasing the demand by left ventricular hypertrophy, and may therefore lead to early, sudden death.

Coarctation

Coarctation varies, anatomically, from a sharply localized narrowing, usually at the point of attachment of the ductus arteriosus, to virtual absence of a length of aortic arch (hypoplastic left heart syndrome). The femoral pulses are weak and delayed relative to the radials, or may be absent unless a patent ductus is feeding the aorta distal to the coarctation, in which case there will be cyanosis of the lower part of the body. There is a systolic murmur well heard over the back. It is usually several years before collateral vessels can be detected clinically or radiologically.

There are very many other congenital heart lesions, and anomalies of the aorta and of the pulmonary veins, of great interest and clinical importance, which may present diagnostic problems. In some of the most severe, murmurs are absent. Specialist help should always be sought sooner rather than later.

General management of children with heart disease

There are two general points relevant to the support given by the doctor to the child with heart disease and his parents; first, the natural anxiety generated by the knowledge (or fear) that the child has a weak heart and second, the question of restrictions on physical activities. Heart disease equates in the public mind with coronaries, blood pressure, strokes and sudden catastrophes. It probably comes second only to mental and nervous disease in its capacity to induce anxiety. The nature of the child's disability should be explained to the parents in terms which they can understand, and with as much optimism as is compatible with truth. They should be assured that the child will not have heart attacks (except in the rare conditions where this is a possibility) and is not in danger of sudden death. If the child's activities do not need to be restricted, this must be emphasized. The likely time for further investigations and the therapeutic possibilities should be outlined. Ignorance breeds anxiety. It will not do to say, 'He has a little heart murmur' and leave it at that. An early specialist opinion will always be appreciated.

Physical activities should not be restricted without good reason. Small VSD's and mild pulmonary stenosis, for example, will not limit cardiac reserve significantly. There is an important difference between competitive activities, in which the determined child may overstretch himself, and non-competitive sports in which he can stop when he tires. The only serious risks are in children with impaired coronary blood flow. Children with congenital heart disease should be given penicillin cover for dental extractions to minimize the risk of subacute bacterial endocarditis.

Further reading

Jordan S.C. & Scott O. (1973) *Heart Disease in Paediatrics*. Butterworth, London.

Chapter 11

THE RESPIRATORY TRACT

The mortality from disorders of the respiratory tract has decreased dramatically in the last 30 years. However, respiratory tract infections remain an important cause of morbidity; they are one of the most common reasons for a child being taken to a doctor or admitted to hospital.

Certain problems are more common at certain ages as shown in Fig. 28. This age variation is not entirely explained by the susceptibility of certain age groups to particular micro-organisms. The same organism may cause different illnesses at different ages; respiratory syncytial virus which commonly causes lower respiratory tract illness (bronchiolitis) in infants, is more likely to cause a cold or a sore throat in older children.

UPPER RESPIRATORY TRACT

Examination of the ears, nose and throat

This is an important part of the general examination of any child, and essential in an ill child. An auriscope is used to examine the ear drums. If wax obscures the view it must be gently removed, with a wax hook or a cotton swab on the end of a wooden applicator stick. If the wax is very hard, softening ear drops may be needed first. Young children dislike having their ears examined, but with practice the procedure is painless. The infant is held by the mother as shown in Fig. 27, her hands ensuring that the child's head is secure, so that the speculum cannot be accidentally rammed into the meatus.

The mouth must be examined thoroughly and the state of the gums, teeth, tongue and buccal mucosa noted as well as the back of the throat. Older children will on request say 'Ah' and reveal the posterior pharynx. For younger children a good view is sometimes obtained by asking the child to put out his tongue. As a last resort a wooden spatula may be needed to depress the tongue. When this is done the child must be held firmly by the mother.

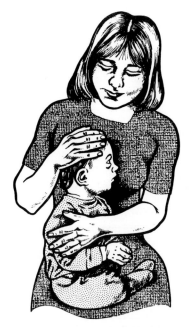

Fig. 27. Mother holding child ready for examination of ears. One hand presses the child's head securely to her chest, the other hand controls the child's outer arm, and presses inwards so trapping the inner arm also.

Acute coryza

The common cold is no more serious in children than in healthy adults. Though mothers are alarmed when their young infants get colds, very few present problems. One possible problem is difficulty with breathing; babies breathe through their nose and if it is blocked may be unable to convert easily to mouth breathing. Further, it is impossible to suck from a feeding bottle and breathe through the mouth at the same time. In these circumstances

decongestant nose drops, for example $\frac{1}{4}\%$ ephedrine, are sometimes given immediately before a feed. A second and more
serious problem is that coryza in an infant may be the precursor
of a lower respiratory tract infection.

Sinusitis

The frontal and sphenoidal sinuses do not develop until 5 and 9
years respectively. The maxillary and ethmoidal sinuses are small
in these years and, in general, sinusitis is uncommon before the
age of 5.

Otitis media

This is common throughout the first 8 years of childhood, and is
generally associated with an infection of the nasopharynx.

In the older child the cardinal symptoms of earache, discharge
or deafness make detection easy. But in infants it may not be so
obvious. They usually have a high fever and are irritable, rolling
their heads from side to side, or rubbing their ears.

At onset there may be just mild inflammation of the pars
flaccida (the superior part of the tympanic membrane) with
dilated vessels running down the handle of the malleus and an
absent light reflex. This progresses to a red bulging tympanic
membrane which may perforate and discharge pus.

Antibiotic therapy is given for a week. The most frequent
pathogens isolated are strep. pneumoniae and haemophilus
influenzae. Below the age of 3 haemophilus is the commonest
pathogen identified, so that ampicillin is the antibiotic of choice.
Aspirin is invaluable for the fever and pain.

Mastoiditis, lateral sinus thrombosis, meningitis, and cerebral
abscess are rare complications. Persistent infection or discharge—
chronic otitis media—is more common.

'*Glue ear*' (secretory otitis media, serous otitis media)

The accumulation of sticky serous material in the middle ear
cavity may arise insidiously or following acute otitis media.
The ear drum is usually dull and retracted. The malleus handle
is more horizontal than usual and appears shorter, broader and

whiter. The light reflex may be absent. There is usually conductive hearing loss. The peak incidence is from 5–9 years when it is the commonest reason for hearing loss. If intensive treatment with antibiotics, antihistamines and decongestant nose drops does not correct the condition, myringotomy and drainage of the middle ear may be needed.

Any child who has otitis media must be followed up until the drum is normal. If response to treatment is slow or infections recur, an ear nose and throat specialist should be consulted.

Deafness

Hearing exists before birth and can be demonstrated in neonates. They startle to a loud noise, or become quiet in response to a diminuendo growl. An infant's hearing is most easily tested at 9 months of age when the child has an insatiable curiosity for new sounds. All children should be tested at this age using the tests described on page 62. Standard pure tone audiometry is not usually possible until the child is 3–4 years old.

Deafness may originate from pre-, peri- or post-natal factors:
1 Prenatal factors include hereditary deafness, maternal infection (e.g. rubella), and congenital atresia of the meatus.
2 Perinatal factors include anoxia and haemorrhage, and kernicterus resulting from haemolytic disease of the newborn.
3 Postnatal factors include meningitis and encephalitis, otitis media, and ototoxic drugs.

If a child has significant deafness the parents complaint will probably be that the child does not talk. In addition the child may have temper tantrums or other behaviour problems.

Most 'deaf' children have some residual hearing, and so will be helped by a hearing aid which can be fitted as early as 3 months of age. That is the start of the treatment, not the end. The parents need to realize that the child has lost a year or so of normal auditory stimulation, and the deficit must be repaid. The child requires prolonged exposure to speech and sounds at a level which he can hear with the hearing aid.

Although the local authority has to provide education for any child over the age of 2 with severe hearing loss, it is only the very severe—totally deaf—who are admitted to special units so early. Most 'deaf' children will enter the 'partially hearing unit' of a nursery school at 3 to 4 and then progress to similar units attached to normal schools or to special schools for the deaf. The teachers of the deaf not only teach the children but perform a valuable role in advising parents before the child enters school.

Tonsils and adenoids

Lymphoid tissue grows rapidly in the first 5 years of life; thereafter the rate of growth decreases. Tonsils and adenoids are usually small in the infant and reach their greatest size relative to body size between 4 and 7. Cervical glands are similarly 'large' during this period, and in response to local infection they enlarge more rapidly and to a greater extent than do those of adults.

Acute tonsillitis

This is very common in the age group 2–8. It is uncommon in infants. There is sudden onset of fever and sore throat. The child often vomits and may have abdominal pains. Both tonsillitis and otitis media are commonly associated with febrile convulsions. The tonsils appear enlarged and fiery red; exudate later appears. The commonest pathogen to be cultured is a beta-haemolytic streptococcus, but no bacterial pathogen can be identified in over half the cases. The presence of small petechiae on the palate or ulcers on the buccal mucosa or gums makes a viral aetiology more likely. Aspirin and plenty of cool drinks provide symptomatic relief. Penicillin is given on the basis that the streptococcus may be the cause. Theoretically a 10-day course of penicillin should be given to prevent rheumatic fever, but unless time is spent explaining this to the parents most will stop giving the penicillin after 3 or 4 days when their child is better.

Complications are uncommon; they may be immediate or delayed.

1 Immediate complications are (a) *Peritonsillar abscess* (quinsy) which is characterized by severe symptoms of tonsillitis and marked dysphagia. The tonsil appears displaced towards the midline with the anterior pillar of the fauces pushed forward. (b) *Cervical abscess*. Marked cervical adenitis is usual at the time of tonsillitis, but occasionally infection localizes in one of the

tonsillar lymph glands to form an abscess. Early antibiotic treatment of peritonsillar or cervical abscess may produce cure, but once they are fully developed surgical drainage is required.
2 Delayed complications after certain streptococcal infections of the tonsil are (a) *Rheumatic fever* (page 167) 1–2 weeks after the infection. (b) *Acute nephritis* (page 188) 2–3 weeks after the infection.

Tonsillectomy

This operation is becoming less fashionable. It is reserved chiefly for children over the age of 4 who have had (1) Recurrent bouts of acute tonsillitis (more than 3 a year), (2) Peritonsillar abscess, or (3) Persistent or chronic infection of the tonsils.

Parents seek the operation for a multiplicity of reasons. They need to be told that in general tonsillectomy does not prevent the child catching colds, sore throats, or bronchitis; it does not improve the child's appetite or growth. Large healthy tonsils rarely cause any trouble—'Large tonsils need to be removed from the text book and not from the child's throat'.

Adenoidectomy

This is usually done at the same time as tonsillectomy. Indications for it to be done independently are recurrent otitis media, sinusitis or nasal obstruction.

Stridor

Stridor is noisy breathing originating from above the bronchi. It commonly originates from the larynx and is mainly inspiratory in timing.

The young child's larynx is not only relatively smaller, but also flabby compared with the firm cartilaginous walls of the adult larynx. It is a voice bag not a voice box and it collapses and obstructs easily.

Congenital stridor

In extreme cases, stridor may be audible from birth. This is uncommon and may be caused by abnormalities of the pharynx, larynx or trachea. The least rare form, 'congenital laryngeal stridor', does not cause complete obstruction and lessens as the child grows though a proportion of the children are found later to have a neurodevelopmental disorder.

This is common from 1–4 years, and alarming. Onset is sudden; stridor develops, the cry is harsh and there is a barking cough (croup) which sounds like a performing seal calling for herrings. There is moderate fever and systemic illness. On examination the fauces are mildly infected, but sometimes the epiglottis can be seen inflamed and like a red cherry as the tongue is depressed (acute epiglottitis). Apart from stridor there may be indrawing of the ribs and suprasternal notch if obstruction is marked. A raised respiratory rate and crepitations or ronchi in the lung fields generally mean that the lower respiratory tract is also involved: laryngo-tracheo-bronchitis.

Viral causes are commonest, but haemophilus influenzae may be the cause, and for that reason ampicillin is given. In hospital the child is put in a humid air tent. Sedation, e.g. promethazine, lessens the child's anxiety and may help the breathing.

Management poses a lot of problems. It is not usually difficult to exclude rare causes of acute respiratory obstruction such as diphtheria, or an abscess, gland or tumour compressing the larynx. Inhalation of a foreign body is more difficult to exclude, particularly if it is not a radio-opaque foreign body. But the most difficult decision is whether to admit the child to hospital. A case can be made for admitting any child with stridor of sudden onset for observation lest total obstruction develops necessitating tracheostomy. In practice admission is usually confined to those whose stridor is associated with one of the following

—acute epiglottitis;

—marked respiratory distress;

—age under 1 year;

—very worried parents.

The stridor usually lessens within 12 hours and has gone within 3 days. If it persists or recurs laryngoscopy is indicated.

Nose bleeds (epistaxes)

The usual site is the anterior inferior corner of the nasal septum (Little's area). The commonest causes are minor injury and upper respiratory tract infections. At the time of such infection the child may alarm everyone by suddenly coughing up or vomiting blood which has been swallowed. In such cases the nose should be examined carefully to identify the source of the blood.

First aid management consists of sitting the child up, leant slightly forward, with a pad of cotton wool to mop up the blood. The child is comforted, told to breathe through the mouth and not to swallow the blood as that tends to cause vomiting.

LOWER RESPIRATORY TRACT

The bronchi and other airways together with the blood vessels supplying them are present by the 20th week of gestation. Thereafter they enlarge but do not reduplicate. In contrast the alveoli and their blood vessels are relatively few in number at birth, and during the first 8 years a period of active production of alveoli raises their number from 20 million to the adult complement of 300 million. One of the problems of respiratory disease in early childhood is that in addition to direct lung damage the disease may interfere with normal lung development.

The airways of an infant are particularly liable to obstruction. A tiny amount of mucus or a small degree of bronchospasm may narrow the airway dangerously leading to poor oxygenation or collapse of a lung segment.

The thoracic cage is more mobile in young children than in adults. In response to airways obstruction the sternum and lower ribs may be sucked in with each inspiration. Accurate timing of the respiratory rate is vital; it rises much more readily than an adult's and reflects the severity of the disorder. Because an infant's breathing is often irregular the rate should be timed over a full minute before the baby is disturbed or undressed. (It is impossible to time a crying infant's respiration.) The respiratory rate in the neonatal period is 30–40/min. By the age of 2 months the rate is under 30/min. A respiratory rate of over 40/min is abnormal and by far the most likely cause is a respiratory infection. However, one needs to remember the other possible causes for a rapid respiratory rate: heart failure, metabolic acidosis, neurological disease and hysterical overbreathing (in adolescents). Tactile vocal fremitus is of little use in children, mainly because their voices make only high frequency sounds. Percussion for dullness or hyper-resonance is very helpful but the usefulness of auscultation of a young child's chest is limited by the fact that the sounds are very freely transmitted making localization difficult. It is important to ensure that coarse crepitations are not in fact noises transmitted from the throat. Bronchial breathing can often be heard over the upper half of a normal child's chest because of direct transmission from the main bronchi.

Bronchitis and bronchiolitis

Acute bronchitis occurs at all ages and is characterized by cough and fever. It is a common early feature of both measles and whooping cough. Chronic bronchitis is very rare in children.

Bronchiolitis is confined to infants. Most cases are caused by respiratory syncytial virus and occur in winter epidemics. Older members of the household merely have mild upper respiratory tract symptoms. Bronchiolitis develops suddenly. In the morning the infant may just be a bit snuffly, but by afternoon he is irritable, coughing and breathless. The respiratory rate is high and as respiratory distress increases cyanosis may appear. Widespread high pitched ronchi and crepitations can be heard throughout the lungs. The infant should be admitted to hospital where intensive care is possible and artificial ventilation available if the dyspnoea worsens. The infants are nursed in extra oxygen and humidity. Antibiotics are often given as it is difficult to distinguish from pneumonia. Nasogastric tube feeding is likely to be needed for the very breathless infant, and careful attention has to be paid to fluid and calorie intake. The crisis lasts for 2–3 days only and then rapid recovery occurs. Up to half the infants who have bronchiolitis caused by respiratory syncytial virus subsequently develop recurrent wheezing.

Pneumonia

Bronchopneumonia

This is commonest in the younger child (Fig. 28), or in an older child who has some chronic condition, e.g. severe cerebral palsy. A wide variety of organisms can be responsible, and in the infant respiratory syncytial virus is the most important. It commonly follows bronchitis, measles and whooping cough.

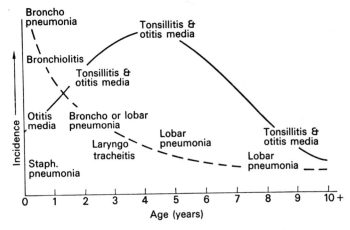

Fig. 28. The incidence of respiratory infections at different ages.

Onset may be sudden or gradual, and fever is also variable. The specific features are rapid breathing and a dry cough (it is unusual for children to spit out sputum—they swallow it). Generalized crepitations and ronchi are present, and although chest X-ray shows small patches of consolidation it is unusual to detect them clinically. Cyanosis occurs in severe cases, and infants may develop secondary cardiac failure.

Hospitalization is needed for the infant and for any child with respiratory distress. At first humidity and oxygen are given. If there are signs of much loose secretions humidity is withheld and physiotherapy becomes more important. A broad spectrum antibiotic is given.

Lobar pneumonia

This afflicts the 4–10 year old child, presenting suddenly with a characteristic picture. The previously healthy school child develops a sudden illness with high fever. There may be pain in the chest or the abdomen or the neck sometimes causing the child to lean towards the affected side. The child is sick and confused. He looks flushed, is breathing fast with an expiratory grunt and is using the alae nasi. There may be a 'cold sore' (herpes simplex) on the lip. The respiratory rhythm may be reversed so that the pause comes after inspiration rather than expiration. There is often no cough. The classical signs of consolidation may not be present at first but repeated examination will usually reveal them. A transient pleural rub is common.

Lobar pneumonia is usually caused by the pneumococcus, and penicillin achieves a speedy recovery. Within 24 hours there is usually dramatic improvement. Provided that the home situation is reasonable this is a safe and rewarding condition to treat at home. The child is dramatically ill, but the mother with the doctor's support can get the child fit and happy fast. In these circumstances it is best to give the initial dose of penicillin by injection as the ill child is likely to vomit medicine. A hypnotic will ensure sleep for the child, and if there is a troublesome cough, a cough suppressant is given. The mother will need to be given general advice about diet: plenty of drinks and not to worry about poor food intake; and advice about the room. Some families ceremonially light the fire in the child's bedroom as soon as the child has a high fever, which is just the time the child wants to be cool.

A child with pneumonia should be afebrile and well a week after onset. If there are still signs or symptoms present, careful examination including chest X-ray should be repeated to exclude such complications as a pleural effusion or lobar collapse.

Staphylococcal pneumonia

This is a severe form of pneumonia which affects infants, and children with fibrocystic disease. It is characterized by lung abscesses on X-ray, and the sudden appearance of empyema or pneumothorax clinically. Prolonged treatment with an antibiotic effective against penicillin-resistant staphylococci is required.

Recurrent respiratory tract infections

Any child who has recurrent lower respiratory tract infections must be fully examined to seek a cause. Investigations should include chest X-ray, sweat electrolytes, immunoglobulin assay, tuberculin test and full blood count. Although many children have this battery of tests it is worth pointing out that recurrent respiratory infections are common, whilst fibrocystic disease is rare and an immunological or white blood cell deficiency extremely rare. Frequently no cause is found and one is left with the conclusion that the child's recurrent problems originate from a combination of hereditary predisposition and an unfavourable environment (e.g. a crowded poor home).

Children aged 4–8 with a persistent or recurrent cough are an even commoner problem. This has usually followed a bout of winter bronchitis, yet the child is still coughing—particularly at night—several months later. It is worth going carefully over the history to decide whether this is a child who is catching frequent upper respiratory tract infections; this is common when the child first goes to nursery or school and meets a lot of new infections. Another reason for persistent cough is that children rarely blow their noses—they have more important things to do—so that mucus may trickle down the back of the pharynx causing the child to cough. Similarly in the older child sinusitis is an important cause of a persistent cough.

Sometimes the history suggests that the initial illness was probably whooping cough. A persistent cough following pertussis is common. In either case both chest X-ray and tuberculin test have a useful therapeutic role as well as excluding pulmonary collapse or tuberculosis.

Usually the parents are disturbed by the nocturnal cough more than the child. Cough suppressants (e.g. codeine) and a sedative (e.g. promethazine) are valuable. Simple measures such as warming a cold bedroom, or cooling a hot one, or giving the child a fruity drink to have by the bed often help.

It is common for asthma to present in early life as recurrent bouts of infection or coughing rather than as obvious wheezing. This will be considered in the next section.

Inhaled foreign bodies

Babies and toddlers are most at risk, for they tend to put everything into their mouths. Older children sometimes accidentally inhale objects during games or whilst stuffing their mouths too full of peanuts or sweets.

A foreign body may lodge at any level. At the time the child will cough, splutter or make choking noises. Then there may be a quiet period of a few days until the impacted object causes a local reaction or a secondary reaction lower down the respiratory tract. In the larynx an object is likely to cause a croupy cough and stridor, in the trachea or large bronchi, a cough and wheeze. Beyond an impacted foreign body the lung, or a lobe of it, may collapse or develop obstructive emphysema.

Whenever the possibility of a foreign body is suspected both antero-posterior and lateral X-rays of the neck and chest should be taken. Translucent objects may not show and the search may have to be continued by direct laryngoscopy and bronchoscopy, which would in any case be required to remove the object.

THE WHEEZY CHILD

Wheezing children are a common and worrying problem. The different diagnostic labels that are applied to them confuse both parents and doctors. Part of the confusion arises from the fact that there is no precise definition of 'asthma', 'wheezy bronchitis', 'allergic bronchitis' or 'asthmatic bronchitis'. Therefore it is best to consider them all as part of the spectrum of the wheezy child. Many infants and children show an exaggerated response to upper respiratory tract infections. At the time of a cold they develop a troublesome cough and ronchi can be heard in the chest. Some children outgrow this phase, but others develop recurrent bouts of wheezing and eventually are diagnosed as having asthma.

Therefore, 'wheezy bronchitis' tends to be used as a label for young children, and 'asthma' for those older children in whom the full clinical pattern emerges. Asthma is characterized by recurrent bouts of wheezing, breathlessness and cough due to intermittent reversible obstruction of the peripheral airways. It tends to occur in response to a variety of stimuli, and most often in children with a personal or family history of allergy.

Many affected children have an elevated serum IgE. Eosinophilia may be present in the peripheral blood, sputum and nasal secretions.

Incidence

Up to 10% of infants have a tendency to wheeze in the first 2 years of life. Most grow out of it. About 3% of school children are considered to have 'asthma' compared with a 1% incidence in adults, which suggests that many outgrow their asthma.

Clinical features

There is often a family history of asthma, eczema or hay fever; and the child may have had, or develop, other hypersensitivity phenomena. Eczema is particularly common from 1–8 years of age and hay fever in the school child.

In the early years the child suffers from recurrent respiratory infections which persists longer than usual. Colds 'go to the chest', coughs persist, and the parents may notice wheezing. The wheezing may steadily worsen for a day or two before gradually improving. As the child becomes older the bouts become more clearly defined and more strikingly intermittent. The onset is sudden, and the child starts wheezing or coughing; breathlessness increases and with it fear. On examination the respiratory rate is increased and the child may be using the accessory muscles of respiration or pushing his hands against a table to force air out in expiration. The wheeze is mainly expiratory and on auscultation prolonged expiratory ronchi are followed by short inspiratory ronchi. Crepitations are variable.

Between attacks there are usually no symptoms or signs. Some children with frequent severe attacks develop hyperinflation, with a barrel-shaped chest, limited chest movement and hyper-resonance. In young children upper respiratory tract infections appear to be the commonest cause, but as the child grows up other precipitating factors may become apparent—specific allergens, exercise, emotional upsets and changes of weather or environment.

MANAGEMENT

The aim is to reduce the frequency of attacks and to make the child and family confident that they can conquer any attack that does occur, without disruption of home or school life. Precipitating factors should always be sought (Fig. 29). Although many of the children produce positive skin reactions to pollens, house dust, and house-dust mite, these tests have to be interpreted in the light of the clinical history for only a few derive benefit from a course of densensitization injections. In all cases it is worth reducing the child's exposure to likely allergens such as house dust and animal dander—pets should be banned from the bedroom, the bedroom 'spring cleaned' regularly, a foam rubber pillow used and a polythene cover put over the mattress. Emotional problems at home or school can often be helped, but it must be realized that asthma generates its own emotional problems for the family; it is a frightening and at times terrifying condition. The concerned and competent doctor can completely change the situation. The family need to know that asthma tends to become less troublesome as the child grows up—that less than a quarter of affected 5-year-olds will be troubled by it at the age of 20. They

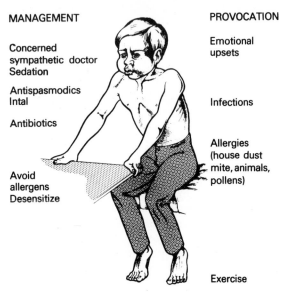

MANAGEMENT

Concerned
sympathetic doctor
Sedation

Antispasmodics
Intal

Antibiotics

Avoid
allergens
Desensitize

PROVOCATION

Emotional
upsets

Infections

Allergies
(house dust
mite, animals,
pollens)

Exercise

Fig. 29. Precipitating features in childhood asthma and possible solutions.

need to know that there are plenty of ways of preventing attacks and even more ways of stopping attacks which the family can employ for themselves. The parents and child need to know that death will not occur during an attack.

In the last 5 years disodium cromoglycate has emerged as a valuable prophylactic agent. It is inhaled as a powder from an 'Intal' spinhaler, twice or thrice daily. It is believed to interfere with the release of spasmogens from mast cells of the bronchial wall. Long term therapy reduces the frequency of asthmatic attacks in a large proportion of children. The introduction of disodium cromoglycate and the occasional use of steroid aerosols has reduced greatly the number of children requiring long term corticosteroid therapy.

TREATMENT OF WHEEZING

A mild attack will often respond to oral antispasmodics such as salbutamol, orciprenaline or ephedrine. The child should be up and about, leading as normal a life as possible, unless feeling really ill and feverish.

More severe attacks require to be stopped faster. Subcutaneous adrenaline or intravenous aminophylline act faster, whilst aminophylline suppositories have the advantage that they can be administered by the parents. Pressurized aerosols containing sympathomimetic drugs are easily used by the patient, but over use tends to occur and can be dangerous. Salbutamol aerosols are probably the safest, but strict instructions must be given and written down to limit the number of 'puffs' used. Whenever asthma appears to have originated from an infection, that infection will require specific therapy. In addition, antibiotics are usually given for severe or prolonged wheezing, if only to prevent secondary infection.

Status asthmaticus describes a state in which severe broncho-spasm has not responded to therapeutic measures, or has lasted for over six hours. It is a dangerous state, and the child should be admitted to hospital. In addition to the antispasmodics, sedatives and antibiotics previously mentioned, corticosteroids may be dramatically effective; it is unusual for them to be needed for more than three days. Oxygen is given to the very breathless or cyanosed child, and in extreme circumstances bronchial lavage may be needed to clear the obstructed airways of sticky secretions and intermittent positive pressure ventilation used. One of the curious features of status asthmaticus is that the act of admission to hospital sometimes stops the attack before any drugs have been given. This seems to be related more to the change in emotional atmosphere than to physical allergenic differences between home and hospital.

Asthma still causes a number of childhood deaths. When it does occur the attack has usually lasted several hours. Apart from mortality, the morbidity needs to be considered. Repeated attacks of asthma may lead to pulmonary complications particularly emphysema and chronic bronchitis. Growth may be restricted particularly if prolonged steroid treatment is needed. Educational and social problems may arise; some children who cannot manage at normal school are admitted to schools for the physically handicapped and delicate, and others to boarding school. This form of 'parentectomy' is reserved for the child who has intractable wheezing in the home environment. Family life can be completely overshadowed by the fact that one child has asthma. This should be rare; asthma is a challenge which the doctor can help the family overcome.

Further reading

Simpson H. (1974) The wheezy child. *British Journal of Hospital Medicine*, **12**, 471.
Forfar J.O. & Arneil G.C. (eds) (1973) Respiratory disorders. Chapter 12, *Textbook of Paediatrics*, Churchill Livingstone, London and Edinburgh.

Chapter 12

THE ALIMENTARY TRACT

Like most childhood illness, alimentary tract disorders are usually acute and infective. These are most serious in infancy, when fluid and electrolyte balance can become dangerously disturbed within a matter of hours and cause death if not recognized and treated. Intestinal obstructions are also important and may be of congenital origin or acquired. Less common, but equally important, are malabsorption states including coeliac disease and cystic fibrosis. In childhood, peptic ulcers, ulcerative colitis and Crohn's disease are uncommon, and neoplasm very rare.

SYMPTOMS AND SIGNS OF ALIMENTARY DISORDERS

The principal symptoms of acute alimentary disease are vomiting, diarrhoea and abdominal pain; of chronic disease, failure to thrive and diarrhoea. Constipation is, of course, a feature of acute intestinal obstruction, but chronic constipation and recurrent abdominal pain are not commonly due to alimentary tract disease. Abdominal distension is a feature of some acute and some chronic disorders.

It is very common for babies to bring up a small amount of food when breaking wind after a feed. This is possetting, a normal process that may be confused with vomiting by an inexperienced mother. Possetting is not accompanied by other symptoms, the baby is happy and gains weight well. Significant vomiting (Table 8) will be accompanied by weight loss, or at least by inadequate weight gain except in over-feeding.

In the same way, the existence of diarrhoea or constipation should not be accepted without detailed enquiry. The number and consistency of stools passed by children, especially infants, is very variable and is influenced by diet. Breast-fed babies pass loose, bright yellow, odourless stools, usually three or four times a day but often after every feed and sometimes as infrequently as once a week. Bottle-fed babies pass paler, firmer, more acid stools

Table 8. Causes of Vomiting

1. Feeding errors
   (a) In infants, too much food, too little food, the wrong kind of food, or faulty feeding technique
   (b) In older children, dietetic indiscretions
2. Infections
   (a) Gastritis (with or without enteritis)
   (b) Parenteral infections (e.g. tonsillitis, meningitis)
   (c) Acute appendicitis
3. Mechanical causes
   (a) Intestinal obstruction, congenital or acquired
   (b) Hiatus hernia: lax oesophagus
4. Raised intracranial pressure
   (a) Meningitis: encephalitis
   (b) Space-occupying lesions (tumour, abscess, haematoma)
5. Metabolic disorders
   (a) Disorders of amino-acid and sugar metabolism
   (b) Adrenal insufficiency
   (c) Ketosis; uraemia
   (d) Intolerance of, or allergy to, food components (e.g. gluten, lactose)
6. Psychological problems
   (a) Periodic syndrome ('cyclical vomiting')
   (b) Rumination
7. Miscellaneous
   (a) Travel sickness
   (b) Migraine
   (c) Poisoning

which smell. If fed on evaporated milk, the consistency and frequency may be similar to that of a breast-fed baby: if fed on dried milk, the stools are usually formed and may be quite hard, causing the baby to strain when defaecating. Unless this straining causes pain or rectal bleeding, or the bowels are being opened less than once a day, this should not be called constipation. Many toddlers and some older children (and some adults) continue to have 3 or 4 bowel actions a day, after meals. If the stool consistency and weight gain are satisfactory, this is not abnormal. Chronic constipation (page 102) may lead to faecal impaction and soiling, which may be mistakenly interpreted as diarrhoea. The principal causes of diarrhoea are shown in Table 9.

Abdominal pain is an important symptom but does not necessarily indicate abdominal disease. Acute central abdominal pain and vomiting are, for example, common symptoms of tonsillitis in young children. Recurrent abdominal pain may be a symptom of emotional stress. From about the age of 2 years

Table 9.   Causes of Diarrhoea

---

1. Feeding errors
   - (a) In infants, too much food, too little or the wrong kind
   - (b) In older children, dietetic indiscretion
2. Inflammatory lesions
   - (a) Enteritis, including dysentery
   - (b) Ulcerative colitis: regional ileitis
   - (c) Lambliasis (giardiasis)
   - (d) Parenteral infections
3. Malabsorption states
   - (a) Steatorrhoea (coeliac disease: cystic fibrosis)
   - b) Disaccharide intolerance

---

children can indicate the site of a pain. In infants, abdominal pain may be inferred from spasms of crying, restlessness and drawing up the knees. It is a very common symptom throughout childhood and is usually of no serious significance. The presence of vomiting, bowel disturbance or fever in association with abdominal pain should prompt a more detailed appraisal, with re-examination after a few hours.

Abdominal distension can be difficult to assess because of the very great normal variation. Fat babies appear to have bigger tummies than thin, muscular babies. Toddlers are normally rather pot-bellied in comparison with older children and coloured children in comparison with white. The mother will usually be able to say whether the abdomen is swollen.

It is important to recognize dehydration and wasting, especially in infants. Clinical dehydration results from inadequate intake (which is not common) or excessive loss by vomiting, diarrhoea or polyuria. The combination of diarrhoea and vomiting, which is necessarily accompanied by inadequate intake, leads to losses of fluid and electrolytes. This is seen in its most dramatic form of infantile gastro-enteritis ('D and V'). The anterior fontanelle and the eyes become sunken, the skin loses its normal elasticity, the infant has an anxious look, a persistent cry and is restless. If the condition progresses, the baby becomes quiet and still, with sunken abdomen and signs of peripheral circulatory failure. In the older child, the lips and tongue become dry, and the eyes a little sunken. After infancy, vomiting rapidly leads to ketosis which is recognized by the smell of the breath and acidotic breathing. Dehydration at any age, if it results from vomiting and/or diarrhoea, will lead to a reduced urinary output: measurement of urine output is therefore helpful when practicable.

Examination of the abdomen

Examination of the abdomen in children requires patience, gentleness and a warm hand. It is helpful for the doctor to get down to the same level as the child by sitting or kneeling, unless the child is on a high bed or couch. This not only makes palpation more satisfactory, it makes conversation easier and the apprehensive child is saved from being towered over. As with older patients, palpation should at first be very gentle, especially if some painful condition is suspected. The right side of the abdomen is sometimes more easily felt from the left side of the patient, either by going round the other side of the cot or by turning the child head to toes. Thus, the liver and the right kidney may be more easily felt. In suspected pyloric stenosis, examination must always be from the left side of the infant.

The liver is normally palpable throughout infancy and early childhood, gradually disappearing under the costal margin in middle childhood. In babies, the edge is usually about 2 cms below the costal margin. The spleen tip is often palpable especially in infants. The kidneys can usually be felt, the right more easily than the left, if the abdomen is reasonably thin and well relaxed. Faecal masses are commonly felt in the line of the colon. Small bowel peristalsis may be visible if the abdominal wall is very thin, as in small pre-term babies and children with wasting diseases.

Rectal examination is rarely omitted by surgeons and often forgotten by physicians. It may be disturbing to young or nervous children, and the decision whether or not to make a rectal examination depends upon what is likely to be learned from it. The doctor is unlikely to detect localized tenderness if the child is crying before he starts. If the patient is an infant or young child with diarrhoea, examination of a stool (as fresh as possible) is often informative. The colour, consistency and smell are noted; the presence of blood or mucus; and the pH noted by testing with paper strips.

The teeth

The ages of usual appearance of the teeth are listed in Appendix 4. There is considerable normal variation in the time of eruption of teeth which may lead to unnecessary worry. The first teeth are sometimes apparent at birth, or no teeth may be cut until after the first birthday. Such extreme variations are usually physiological and only exceptionally due to disease.

It is good practice for the doctor to include the teeth in his examination of the mouth. It gives an opportunity for either congratulation or health education, and occasionally an unexpected alveolar abscess is found to explain a persistent fever or ill health.

Stomatitis

In infancy, stomatitis is usually due to *Candida albicans* (monilia; thrush). This may develop in any baby whose feeds, bottles, teats or dummy have not been adequately sterilized; in babies who have been given broad-spectrum antibiotics, even for a few days only; and in emaciated and very ill infants. It appears as tiny white flecks inside the cheeks, on the tongue and on the roof of the mouth. The only possible source of diagnostic confusion is milk curds which stick to the mouth after feeds. These are usually larger than thrush lesions, and can easily be detached with a spatula. Candida albicans will be cultured in large numbers from a swab (but it should be noted that this organism can often be cultured from the mouths or throats of healthy children). Treatment is aimed first at the cause (correction of faulty sterilization techniques or review of antibiotic policy) and second at elimination of the organism by the local application of nystatin or (in nystatin-resistant cases) amphotericin B. Gentian violet, although cheap and often effective, is extremely messy and makes it difficult to judge progress. It is important to continue local application for a few days after apparent cure, otherwise recurrence is likely.

Candida albicans may also infect the skin of the napkin area (page 176), and exceptionally it may cause systemic infection in children with immunological deficiencies or debilitating diseases.

In older children, stomatitis is usually due to a first infection with herpesvirus hominis. *Herpetic stomatitis* is most common in toddlers, and the lesions are most marked on the lips and tongue. There are vesicles, ulcers and scabs and the condition is painful. The gums are inflamed. There is cervical adenitis. Because of the pain the child will not eat and is often reluctant even to drink. There is general misery, listlessness and a low-grade fever. It is quite exceptional for the infection to spread to any other part of the body. The condition is self-limiting: the discomfort eases after a few days, and the lesions have healed in 2 weeks. Admission to hospital may be necessary to maintain fluid intake, but local applications are of doubtful value and antibiotics should be avoided. Sometimes there is marked enlargement of the cervical glands with oedema of the neck which may raise the spectre of 'Vincent's angina', but unless the relevant organisms can be demonstrated, antibiotics should be withheld. If they are given, the usual consequence is a superadded infection with Candida albicans.

Herpangina

This is the term given to upper respiratory infections associated with ulcers which are confined to the posterior pharynx and fauces. The usual causes are viruses of the Coxackie A group. In some children the ulcers are associated with vesicles on the hands, feet and buttocks—'Hand, Foot and Mouth Disease'.

HERNIAS

Hernias in children may involve the umbilicus, the diaphragm, the inguinal or femoral regions. They differ in some important ways from the hernias of adults.

Umbilical hernia

This is common and harmless. There is a small, sharply defined, circular defect in the centre of the umbilicus through which protrudes a small loop of bowel. Umbilical hernia is always easily reducible and virtually never strangulates. Spontaneous cure is usual before the first birthday. Treatment is not required although adhesive strapping may support the mother's morale. Babies with umbilical hernias may cry (as may babies without hernias) but the hernia should not be regarded as the cause of the crying. In paraumbilical hernia, the orifice is usually immediately above the centre of the umbilicus. This may not heal spontaneously, and surgical repair will be required before the child starts school. Umbilical hernia is an almost constant feature of cretinism, and in this condition the hernia may be quite large. It heals when the cretinism is treated with thyroxin.

Diaphragmatic hernia

The most serious type of diaphragmatic hernia causes difficulties from the moment of birth and results from the failure of one or other leaf of the diaphragm (rarely both) to develop. It is more common on the left side. The lung on the side of the hernia is usually grossly underdeveloped. The hemithorax contains abdominal viscera, the heart is displaced to the opposite side, and the contralateral lung is compressed by the mediastinum. There is, therefore, grave respiratory difficulty from the moment of birth. If the hernia is left-sided, examination reveals the heart beat on the right side of the chest; if on the right, the apex beat is in the left axilla. Percussion note and air entry may be abnormal, but it is unusual to hear bowel sounds except with small hernias that gradually develop over a few days. A chest radiograph makes the diagnosis clear. Early intubation and positive pressure insufflation are usually necessary to maintain life until surgical repair can be undertaken.

Hiatus hernia associated with congenital short oesophagus is more common but less serious. It presents with vomiting in early infancy, sometimes in the neonatal period. There may be a small amount of fresh or altered blood in the vomitus. The vomiting is not as a rule projectile, and weight gain is usually maintained. The diagnosis may be confirmed radiologically by giving a contrast meal. A small knuckle of stomach can be demonstrated above the diaphragm. In the head-down (Trendelenberg) position, oesophageal reflux can be demonstrated, but reflux can occur without hiatus hernia. This condition is usually more of a nuisance than a worry, and conservative management is indicated. This consists of nursing the baby in the sitting position in a baby seat, thickening milk feeds, and introducing solid foods as early as possible. Remission of symptoms can be anticipated towards the end of the first year of life. Exceptionally, the hernia is large and associated with copious vomiting and weight loss. In these cases, surgical repair is required.

Inguinal hernia

This is common in boys, rare in girls. It is often bilateral. A big hernia will form a large swelling in the scrotum, which can be reduced quite easily if the baby is quiet. A small hernia will cause a swelling in the groin which may only be visible intermittently. The smaller the hernia, the more liable it is to strangulate. The doctor should therefore be more concerned about the hernia he cannot see than the one he can. In either case, the danger is present and spontaneous cure is not to be anticipated. Surgical repair should be undertaken at the first convenient moment.

INTESTINAL OBSTRUCTION

Intestinal obstruction may be present at birth, usually as a consequence of malformations of the alimentary tract, or may develop at any age thereafter. The cardinal symptoms are vomiting, abdominal distension, constipation, and (in children old enough to make their feelings clear) pain. Vomiting will lead to fluid and electrolyte loss with clinical signs of dehydration, and later to circulatory failure. Successful treatment therefore depends upon early diagnosis, adequate pre-operative correction of fluid and electrolyte loss, and skilled surgery.

1 In the newborn

The level of the obstruction in the newborn may be anywhere from the oesophagus to the anus. Because swallowing by the fetus is one of the normal routes of disposal of amniotic fluid, obstruction

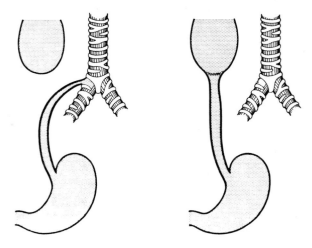

Fig. 30. Tracheo-oesophageal fistula before and after surgical correction.

may lead to accumulation of excess fluid (polyhydramnios) before birth, thus providing a diagnostic clue. The higher the level of obstruction, the more likely is this to occur. It is therefore common with oesophageal atresia but rare with rectal atresia. (Stenosis indicates narrowing of a passage: atresia indicates complete obstruction.) *Oesophageal atresia* is usually associated with tracheo-oesophageal fistula (Fig. 30) so that the bowel is soon filled with air via the fistula. In the absence of a fistula, the bowel remains airless and the abdomen sunken. Because swallowing is impossible, mucus tends to accumulate in the pharynx, and the infant after birth needs frequent aspiration of secretions. True vomiting is impossible, as food cannot reach the stomach, but if feeding is attempted, there will be immediate regurgitation and inhalation of feeds, with choking and cyanosis. Milk in the lungs causes severe pneumonia, and diagnosis should be made before feeding. If there has been polyhydramnios, or if suspicions are aroused by excess secretions, a naso-gastric tube should be passed to demonstrate patency of the oesophagus. If this proves impossible, radiography after the careful instillation of a few mls of contrast medium into the oesophageal pouch will confirm the diagnosis and demonstrate the level of the obstruction. Early diagnosis and skilled surgery offer the best chance of cure, but there are other severe defects in about half the cases. Oeso-phageal and rectal atresia sometimes occur in the same baby.

Atresias at lower levels will cause vomiting and distension. If the obstruction is high, vomiting will be early. The vomit will contain bile because the obstruction is usually below the ampulla of Vater. Distension will be mainly epigastric. If the obstruction is lower, the vomiting will start a little later and the distension will be more generalized. *Duodenal atresia* and stenosis are particularly common in mongols. *Rectal atresia* is usually associated with fistula between the rectum and some part of the genito-urinary tract. An infant with low, complete obstruction cannot pass meconium, but small quantities may be passed by those with high obstruction. In *Hirschsprung's disease*, obstruction is incomplete and is due to a narrow, aganglionic segment of bowel, most commonly in the recto-sigmoid region. *Meconium ileus* is a manifestation of cystic fibrosis. In *malrotation*, the bowel has become twisted at the time of reduction of the normal umbilical hernia of embryonic life and obstruction results from peritoneal bands. There are many other causes of congenital obstruction, and often the precise anatomical diagnosis can only be made at operation. The site of obstruction can often be deduced from the distribution of intestinal gas seen on a straight radiograph taken with the baby vertical. If there is imperforate anus or low rectal atresia, a radiograph is taken with the baby inverted and a metal marker over the anal dimple: the distance from the terminal gas shadow to the marker indicates the depth at which the bowel ends.

2 At later ages

Intestinal obstruction at later ages may be caused by intussusception, pyloric stenosis, volvulus, strangulated inguinal hernia or other rarer causes. *Intussusception* occurs most commonly in infancy. It has been suggested that the change to a mixed diet leads to a change in intestinal flora and that this causes hypertrophy of Peyer's patches, one of which may form the apex of an intussusception. There is also evidence to suggest that viral infections of the bowel may play a role in causation. The infant cries intermittently with colicky abdominal pain, and between attacks is quiet and pale. The spasms become more frequent and more severe, red blood may be passed with a rather loose stool ('red-currant jelly'), and distension and vomiting soon develop. Gentle palpation, preferably while the infant is asleep between attacks of pain, will often reveal a firm, sausage-shaped mass lying somewhere in the line of the colon, often in the upper right quadrant. Rarely, the apex may be felt on rectal examination. In cases of diagnostic difficulty, a contrast enema, given with care, may show the intussusception, and on occasion may cause its reduction. However, the treatment of choice is reduction at open operation, after correction of fluid and electrolyte balance, with resection of any gangrenous bowel.

Pyloric stenosis

Congenital pyloric stenosis is a relatively common condition, the cause of which is still unknown. The marked preponderance in males (about sevenfold), the increased incidence in co-twins, and in close relatives, suggest that there is a genetic contribution to the disorder. On the other hand, it is almost never found in stillborn babies, or babies dying within a few days of birth, and it is therefore arguable whether it should be called 'congenital'. The pathology is a hypertrophy of the circular muscle of the pylorus which leads to progressive obstruction. The onset of symptoms is usually gradual, beginning in the second or third week of life, though occasionally much later. Vomiting is initially slight and intermittent but becomes more frequent, more copious and more forceful (projectile vomiting). Weight gain, which has usually been satisfactory before the onset of symptoms, falls off, eventually stops, and is followed by weight loss. The motions become more and more constipated. Appetite remains ravenous, but if diagnosis is delayed wasting and dehydration follow (Fig. 31). Pyloric stenosis is diagnosed by watching the infant feed. A mass may be felt in the pyloric region before the feed begins, but is often more evident after the feed has been vomited. It is

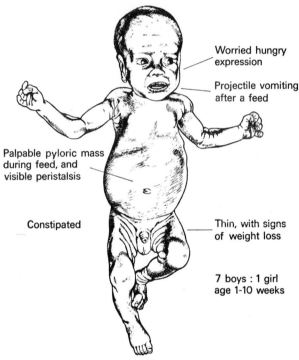

Worried hungry expression

Projectile vomiting after a feed

Palpable pyloric mass during feed, and visible peristalsis

Constipated

Thin, with signs of weight loss

7 boys : 1 girl age 1-10 weeks

Fig. 31. Pyloric stenosis.

the shape and size of a large olive, very firm, and may be felt contracting intermittently. As the stomach fills, waves of peristalsis become visible, crossing the epigastrium from left to right. Gastric peristalsis tends to become more and more marked until the infant vomits, when the vomitus may shoot out several feet. If there is diagnostic difficulty, a contrast meal will show a distended stomach, and a narrow, elongated pyloric canal. The treatment of choice is surgical, the pyloric muscle being divided along its entire length until the mucosa bulges up into the incision · (Ramstedt's operation). Success depends upon adequate preoperative preparation, skilled surgery and anaesthesia, and careful postoperative management. If for any reason surgical treatment cannot be carried out, the condition can be treated medically by giving antispasmodics (atropine methyl nitrate or scopolamine methyl nitrate) shortly before each feed. Medical treatment has to be continued for weeks or months, after which the condition resolves. It is therefore tedious, and weight gain may remain unsatisfactory.

INFECTIVE DIARRHOEA

Acute, infective diarrhoea is common, it spreads rapidly through a closed community like a home or a hospital ward, and it is potentially lethal, especially in the very young. The cause may be viral or bacterial, and a similar illness may result from the ingestion of bacterial exotoxins or chemical poisons. Bacterial infections in the newborn and young infants are most commonly due to one of the many pathological strains of E. Coli: in older children, infections with Salmonella and Shigella organisms predominate.

The most serious symptoms are those due to disturbances of fluid and electrolyte balance resulting from the outpouring of fluid into the alimentary tract. Sometimes this occurs with such rapidity that the infant has become profoundly ill, with clear evidence of fluid loss, before the first loose stool has been passed. Vomiting is commonly present as well, increasing fluid loss and preventing its replacement by the oral route. In the very young there may be fever and leucocytosis, suggesting systemic spread of the infection. In these infants, the administration of appropriate antibiotics is probably helpful. In older children with Salmonella and Shigella infections, antibiotics are disappointing, and indeed there is evidence to suggest that their use may delay clearing of the pathogens from the bowel. The basis of treatment is the correction and maintenance of fluid and electrolyte balance. Mild cases may be treated at home by giving small volumes of clear fluids at frequent intervals for 24 hours followed by gradual re-introduction of milk. Moderate and severe cases require an intravenous drip until oral fluids can be retained, and strict barrier nursing to prevent the spread of infection to others.

MALABSORPTION STATES

In children, malabsorption equates closely with steatorrhoea. There are conditions in which the digestion and absorption of sugars is abnormal, and protein-losing enteropathy occurs very rarely, but fatty diarrhoea occurs much more frequently. Again, there are many possible causes of fatty diarrhoea, but in practice it usually turns out to be due to either coeliac disease or cystic fibrosis of the pancreas. In both conditions the stools are offensive, pale and bulky as well as frequent, and sometimes the mother reports difficulty in flushing them down the toilet because of their tendency to float. Weight gain is unsatisfactory, or there may be frank weight loss with muscle wasting. This contrasts with the big abdomen which is due predominantly to gaseous distension of the bowel. Because the appearance of the stool may be misleading (in either direction), it is essential to measure faecal fat output before diagnosing steatorrhoea. Neither complicated fat balances nor radio-active materials are necessary. A collection is made of faeces corresponding to a food intake of a few days (usually five) and the total fat content determined. A carmine marker is given by mouth at the beginning and end of the five-day period as the corresponding faeces may be passed over a different number of days. The daily average faecal fat content in infants does not as a rule exceed 2–3 grams, or in older children 5 grams. If larger quantities are being excreted, it is probable that the child has coeliac disease or cystic fibrosis. In view of the difficulty of collecting reliable 5 day faecal samples and the need for jejunal biopsy in the diagnosis of coeliac disease, this investigation is falling out of favour in paediatrics.

Coeliac disease

Coeliac disease is the result of a sensitivity to the gluten fraction of wheat, rye or other cereals. Therefore, symptoms are not to be expected before the introduction of cereals into the diet. There is evidence to suggest that the earlier introduction of cereals has led to an increased incidence of coeliac disease. Infants do not need cereals before 4 months of age. In addition to the fatty diarrhoea, wasting and abdominal distension described above, the appetitite is usually very poor and the child is miserable. Many of the children have a fair complexion and long eyelashes (Fig. 32). Sometimes the disease begins acutely, and in these children vomiting may be more conspicuous than diarrhoea: indeed,

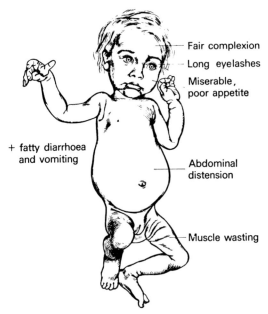

Fair complexion

Long eyelashes

Miserable, poor appetite

+ fatty diarrhoea and vomiting

Abdominal distension

Muscle wasting

Fig. 32. Coeliac disease.

the combination of vomiting and abdominal distension may suggest intestinal obstruction.

There is an enormous range of investigations to which the child suspected of having coeliac disease may be subjected. The diagnosis should not be made without jejunal biopsy, which shows sub-total villous atrophy (a flat appearance). Therefore it is arguable that no other test is necessary. However, there are many children in whom the diagnosis is more of a possibility than a probability, and in such cases alternative tests may be accepted as adequate to exclude the diagnosis. Total faecal fat excretion over a 4–5 day period may be measured, but is valueless unless the collection of stools is complete and accurate. A xylose absorption test, in which a single estimation of blood xylose is made one hour after a loading dose of oral xylose, seems more informative in children than the conventional xylose tolerance test. Small bowel contrast meal may also be helpful.

Treatment consists of exclusion of wheat and rye gluten, and others if necessary. There is usually a rapid and dramatic effect on appetitite and temperament, followed by a good weight gain, but some children do not show improvement until they have been on their diet for 3 or 4 weeks. A few children with coeliac disease also have a temporary intolerance of lactose and do not improve until this has also been eliminated from the diet. Iron-deficiency anaemia is common (megaloblastic anaemia less common), and the rapid growth that follows treatment may precipitate rickets. Iron and vitamin supplements are therefore indicated in the early stages of treatment. Although it is often possible for a coeliac child to return to a normal diet in later childhood without a recurrence of diarrhoea, experience has shown that growth tends to suffer. The diet should therefore be strictly followed at least until growth is complete. On a normal diet, symptoms may recur at any time in adult life ('idiopathic steatorrhoea'), in which case dietetic restrictions are needed again.

Cystic fibrosis (Fibrocystic disease of the pancreas; Muco-viscidosis)

Cystic fibrosis is a serious disease which affects about one child in every 2–3,000 amongst white races. In this ethnic group, it is the commonest disease caused by an autosomal recessive gene. The fundamental defect has not yet been determined, but concerns transport across cell membranes. The symptoms of the disease, though varied, are largely attributable to the secretion of abnormally viscid mucus (mucoviscidosis). The most helpful laboratory test demonstrates increased concentrations of sodium and chloride in sweat, saliva and other body secretions.

Cystic fibrosis may present clinically
1 as intestinal obstruction in the newborn;

154

2 as failure to thrive with fatty diarrhoea, or
3 with recurrent respiratory infections.

In the newborn baby, the meconium may be so glutinous because of the viscid mucus in it that normal peristaltic waves cannot shift it (meconium ileus). Small amounts of meconium

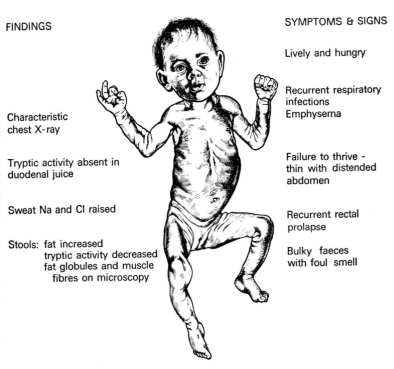

FINDINGS

Characteristic
chest X-ray

Tryptic activity absent in
duodenal juice

Sweat Na and Cl raised

Stools: fat increased
         tryptic activity decreased
         fat globules and muscle
         fibres on microscopy

SYMPTOMS & SIGNS

Lively and hungry

Recurrent respiratory
infections
Emphysema

Failure to thrive -
thin with distended
abdomen

Recurrent rectal
prolapse

Bulky faeces
with foul smell

Fig. 33. Cystic fibrosis.

may be passed; generalized abdominal distension develops over 24–48 hours, and vomiting develops at the same time. An X-ray of the erect abdomen shows evidence of obstruction. At operation there is often obstruction at several sites, and clearing the viscid meconium may be very difficult. The bowel may have to be opened in several places, and washouts with mucolytic agents may be helpful. Unfortunately, even if the obstruction is overcome, the underlying disease remains. Prolapse of the rectum may occur in newborns with cystic fibrosis.

If affected infants pass through the neonatal period without illness, they are likely to present later in infancy because of offensive diarrhoea, poor weight gain, respiratory infections, or combinations of these symptoms. Malabsorption is chiefly due to blockage of the pancreatic ducts by viscid secretions and consequent deficiency of pancreatic enzymes. The diarrhoea may start any time from birth, and is not related to changes in diet. Distension and weight loss resemble those seen in coeliac disease, but the appetite often remains good and the temperament less miserable than in coeliac disease (Fig. 33). Recurrent bronchitis and pneumonia (especially staphylococcal) may begin in infancy or may be delayed for several years. A few children suffer more from sinusitis and nasal polyposis than from chest infections.

Laboratory diagnosis rests chiefly on the demonstration of raised sodium and chloride levels (over 60 mmol/L) in the sweat. Localized sweating is induced by iontophoresis with pilocarpine, and either the sweat is tested in situ by application of an appropriate electrode, or it is absorbed onto filter paper and analysed chemically. The test is not reliable in very young babies, but thereafter is remarkably specific. (Some mothers notice that the baby tastes salty when kissed.) Examination of stools for pancreatic enzymes and undigested food residues may be helpful; examination of duodenal juice is more trouble but more valuable.

Treatment of the pancreatic disorder is relatively simple and consists in the provision of enzymes in powder or tablet form to be taken with food, together with supplements of iron and fat-soluble vitamins initially. The respiratory problems tend to become slowly but progressively worse, and death results from extensive bronchiectasis and cor pulmonale. Therapy is aimed at prevention of chest infections and depends upon physiotherapy and chemotherapy. The pros and cons of chemoprophylaxis are not yet entirely resolved, and the value of small droplet humidification (mist therapy) is still uncertain. In addition to direct treatment of the disease, progressive disability may demand education at a school for the physically handicapped; the parents require genetic counselling; and the family needs continuing support through a long, demanding, and at times distressing illness.

Disaccharide intolerance

Intolerance of disaccharides, notably lactose, may occur in children under the following circumstances:

1 As a temporary complication of steatorrhoea in coeliac disease or cystic fibrosis.

2 As a temporary complication of gastro-enteritis (or other infections).

3 Permanently, as a result of deficiency of lactase, usually genetically determined.

The condition causes a fermentative diarrhoea. It is diagnosed by demonstrating disaccharides in the stools, which are acid; deficiency of disaccharidases in jejunal biopsy specimens; and a good clinical response to the exclusion of the offending sugar. If the intolerance is temporary, lactose may be cautiously reintroduced once recovery from the underlying cause is complete.

Note: Although children with galactosaemia (page 219) cannot tolerate lactose, the lesion is not in the alimentary tract and the disease is not usually classified as an intolerance.

OTHER ALIMENTARY DISORDERS

Food allergy

True allergy to foods is not nearly so common as is often supposed but does occasionally happen. The food proteins most often associated with allergy are cow's milk albumin and the proteins of fish, shellfish and some fruits (strawberries are most notorious). Symptoms of food allergy include vomiting, diarrhoea and abdominal pain; urticarial, erythematous or eczematous rashes; and exceptionally acute anaphylactic symptoms. The diagnosis is supported by appropriate skin tests and confirmed by relief of symptoms when the offending food is excluded, and recurrence when it is re-introduced.

Ulcerative colitis and regional ileitis

Neither of these conditions is common in childhood, and they do not differ in essentials from the adult pattern. Ulcerative colitis most commonly presents with chronic or recurrent bloody diarrhoea with weight loss. Regional ileitis (Crohn's disease) most commonly presents with obstructive symptoms. In the diagnosis of both conditions a barium enema is helpful. In neither disease is the cause understood, so treatment is empirical and not very satisfactory. Physicians modify the diet and prescribe steroids; surgeons resect the offending part; neither lays extravagant claims to success.

Acute abdominal pain

Appendicitis

This occurs at all ages but is uncommon under the age of 2. The most constant features are pain, vomiting, fever and a coated tongue. The diagnosis is usually made on the basis of localized tenderness. With appendix abscess, the history is longer and there is a palpable, tender mass. Diagnostic difficulties may be caused in one direction by an appendix in an unusual position, and in the other by conditions presenting with acute abdominal pain and vomiting. Toddlers with tonsillitis often complain of pain in the abdomen and not in the throat. Their abdominal tenderness is usually generalized or central, but may be maximal in the right iliac fossa. (Warning: Tonsillitis and appendicitis can occur together.)

In acute pyelonephritis the tenderness is usually in the loins. Microscopy of the urine gives the diagnosis. In right lower lobe pneumonia there may be referred pain and tenderness in the right iliac fossa. The respiratory rate will be raised, there are usually abnormal signs in the chest, and a chest X-ray is helpful. Mesenteric adenitis is most confidently diagnosed at laparotomy, when enlarged, inflamed glands and normal appendix are found. The condition may be suspected clinically if the child is more tender than ill and if enlarged glands can be felt. However, once an inflamed appendix perforates and peritonitis supervenes, the prognosis becomes worse. If in doubt 'look and see' is wiser than 'wait and see'.

Giardiasis and worms

Giardia lamblia is a protozoon which commonly inhabits the alimentary canals of children without disturbing their health. Occasionally it causes disease, and this usually takes the form of chronic diarrhoea with semi-formed, khaki-coloured stools and very little constitutional upset. Rarely, infection is associated with steatorrhoea and a clinical picture resembling coeliac disease. The cysts may be identified in the stools, although their presence does not establish that they are causing disease. Treatment is with mepacrine or metranidazole.

Intestinal worms are now seen far less commonly than they used to be. *Threadworms* (Enterobius vermicularis) are relatively common. They cause no symptoms apart from peri-anal itching which may disturb sleep. Diagnosis is made by seeing the worms on the peri-anal skin or stool, or by demonstrating ova from the peri-anal region, best achieved by the use of cellophane swabs or sellotape. Piperazine is the drug of choice, often given as a single dose combined with standardized senna. Apparent failure is usually due to re-infection. Success is then often achieved by treating the whole family, including parents.

The *roundworm* (Ascaris lumbricoides) is uncommon. There are usually no symptoms before a worm is passed with the stools. Piperazine is the drug of choice. *Tapeworms* (Taenia saginata and T. solium) are now exceedingly rare because of high standards of butchering and domestic cooking. They present with the passage of segments. Treatment may be difficult. Niclosamide is probably the drug of choice.

Rectal bleeding

Blood in the stools is always an alarming symptom, although the cause is often trivial. Bleeding from the duodenum or above will usually cause melaena, although copious bleeding (e.g. swallowed blood after epistaxis or tonsillectomy) may cause red blood to appear with the stool. Blood from the ileum or colon is freely mixed with faecal matter: that from the rectum or anus is only on the surface of the stool. If rectal bleeding is associated with painful defaecation, the likely cause is an anal fissure. If a fissure is seen, rectal examination would be very painful and should be avoided.

Many of the commoner causes of rectal bleeding in adults (e.g. piles, rectal carcinoma) do not occur in children. The main causes in childhood are shown in Table 10.

Table 10. Causes of Rectal Bleeding

Site	Condition	Clinical picture
Ileum	Intussusception	Colicky pain: red-current jelly stool: palpable mass
	Bleeding Meckel's diverticulum	Intermittent abdominal pain and bleeding (red or melaena)
Colon	Dysentery (Shigella, Salmonella)	Acute mucoid diarrhoea and pain
	Ulcerative colitis	Mucoid diarrhoea; onset sometimes acute
	Intussusception	
Rectum	Polyp	Recurrent bleeding: no pain
	Prolapse	Prolapse visible
Anus	Fissure	On defaecation, much pain and little blood
	Constipation	

Further reading

Forfar J.O. & Arneil G.C. (1973) Disorders of the alimentary tract. Chapter 11, *Textbook of Paediatrics*. Churchill Livingstone, London and Edinburgh.

Chapter 13

THE SKELETAL SYSTEM

STRUCTURAL VARIATION AND CONGENITAL
ABNORMALITIES

The normal flat-footed baby becomes a bow-legged toddler and
then a knock-kneed primary school child before growing into a
graceful adolescent (Fig. 34).

Flat Feet (pes planus)

A baby has little or no visible plantar arch, and the early foot-
prints confirm this. By the age of 6 the arch should have developed.

Bow Legs (genu varum)

Bow legs are commonest from 0–2 years. The knees may be
$\frac{1}{2}$–1 in. apart when the feet are together; the toes point medially.
If the degree of bowing is gross, rickets should be excluded.

Knock knees (genu valgum)

This is most apparent at 3–4 years of age. When the knees are
together the medial malleoli may be up to $2\frac{1}{2}$ in. apart. Knock
knees persist for longer in the obese child. By the age of 12 the
legs should be straight.

Scoliosis

A lateral curve of the spine is commonly seen in babies, and may
be associated with skull asymmetry (plagiocephaly). Generally

it is a postural scoliosis which goes when the baby is suspended and which has completely gone by the age of 2. Postural scoliosis is seen again at adolescence when it is commoner in girls; when the girl is asked to bend forward the curve straightens out. Fixed scoliosis at any age is likely to mean a vertebral or neurological abnormality.

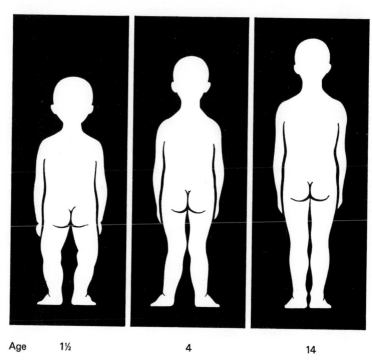

| Age | 1½ | 4 | 14 |

Fig. 34. Normal variation of legs with age.

Talipes (club foot)

Minor degrees of talipes are common at birth, resulting from mechanical pressure in utero. The commonest deviation is that in which there is plantar flexion (equinus) and foot inversion (varus) at the midtarsal joint (Fig. 35). If the foot with talipes equino-varus can be fully dorsiflexed and everted so that the little toe touches the outside of the leg without undue force, it can be expected to correct itself with time. If it cannot be so over-corrected urgent splintage or surgery is needed. The sooner treatment is begun the better the outcome. Talipes calcaneo-valgus describes the dorsiflexed foot which is everted so that the foot lies against the outer border of the leg with the little toe almost touching it. Usually the position is easily corrected by simple exercises.

Congenital defects of the spinal cord such as spina bifida cystica are commonly associated with severe talipes.

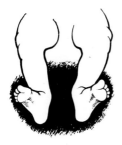
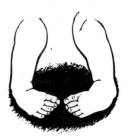

Talipes calcaneo-valgus   Talipes equino-varus

Fig. 35. Talipes.

Congenital dislocation of the hip

Dislocated hips are associated with joint laxity and acetabular dysplasia. Postural factors play a role in their causation. They are commoner in:
—girls;
—babies presenting by the breech;
—full-term rather than pre-term babies;
—the left hip.

Diagnosis is made by specifically testing the hips: a modification of Ortolani's manoeuvre is one such test (Fig. 36). The baby is laid on its back with the feet towards the examiner. The legs are straightened. Then the examiner grasps the child's legs placing the middle finger of each hand on the outer aspects of each hip, and the thumb on the inner side. In turn each hip is half abducted and the leg is lifted up with the middle finger. A dislocated hip

163

slips into the socket with a click. The dislocated hip does not abduct as fully as the normal hip. X-ray examination is unreliable in the first month.

One in 60 babies is found to have hip instability at birth. 85% recover spontaneously, but the remainder persist and may not be detected until the 2-year-old is noticed to have a limp. Early splinting is successful within 2 months in most neonates; but treatment of those detected late is more traumatic and less successful.

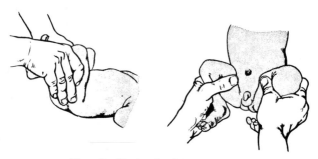

Fig. 36. Testing for dislocation of hips.

Osteogenesis imperfecta

This is a rare condition characterized by fragile bones and lax ligaments. In severe cases multiple fractures occur in utero, whilst milder cases may merely incur a few fractures between the ages of 4 and 14. Familial inheritance is common; affected children may have blue sclerotics and suffer deafness in adult life.

OSTEOMYELITIS (Osteitis)

Pyogenic infection of bone is commoner in children than adults, and in boys than girls.

The usual site is the metaphysis of one of the long bones particularly in the legs. At all ages except infancy staphylococcus aureus is by far the commonest pathogen. The sources of infection and portal of entry are uncertain.

It may present acutely with a high fever and localized pain. An infant may merely refuse to use the affected arm or leg. The cardinal sign of osteomyelitis is a localized point of acute bone tenderness. Over this there may be redness or oedema. There is a neutrophil leukocytosis. Blood culture usually identifies the organism responsible. X-ray is normal at first; it is only after 2 or more weeks that the signs of rarefaction and periosteal new bone formation are seen.

Osteomyelitis is a most serious condition in which the future growth of the bone is in jeopardy. Intensive treatment in hospital is needed. Large doses of antibiotics are given, and it is best to use an antibiotic which is effective against penicillin resistant staphylococci, e.g. lincomycin or fusidic acid.

If treatment is given early complete resolution occurs in most cases. If diagnosis is delayed surgical drainage is more likely to be needed.

Chronic osteomyelitis may result from late or inadequate treatment of acute osteomyelitis or trauma. There is persistent dull bone pain. X-ray shows necrotic areas of bone; it is these areas which harbour the bacteria. Sometimes pus and bone fragments are discharged through the skin to form a fistula. Radical surgery to remove necrotic tissue is combined with systemic antibiotics.

ARTHRITIS

Arthritis is characterized by a painful inflamed joint in which there is limitation of movement in all directions. Swelling is not always present. The joint itself is usually painful but occasionally the pain is referred to another area; hip pain may be referred to the knee.

The more important causes vary with age:

1 Trauma, particularly in the school child. 'Observation hip' refers to a transient hip pain which subsides completely when the child is rested and given analgesics. Preceding trauma is suspected to be the cause, though certain evidence of it is not always obtained.

2 Acute suppurative arthritis—either blood borne or secondary to adjacent osteomyelitis. This occurs mainly in infants and is treated with aspiration, antibiotics and splintage.

3 Henoch–Schönlein syndrome, rheumatic fever and the collagen diseases (see Chapter 14).

4 Any viral infection, particularly rubella and infectious mononucleosis.

5 Septicaemia, particularly with meningococcus, salmonella, shigella and brucella.

6 Tuberculosis, secondary spread having occurred from a pulmonary lesion, and affecting children under 5.

7 Serum sickness and generalized allergic reactions.

8 Haemophilia and Christmas disease. Bleeding into joints is common, and the painful haemarthrosis mimics an acute arthritis.

OSTEOCHONDRITIS AND EPIPHYSITIS

These terms are applied to bone changes which occur, particularly in epiphyses of children, as a result of avascular necrosis or excessive strain on a growing bone. They present as bone pain, with local swelling and tenderness. There is limitation of movement and adjacent muscle wasting. Those that occur in weight bearing joints are the most important, as permanent damage may occur. The best example is Perthes' disease which affects the femoral head of children (usually boys) aged 5–8 years. It causes hip pain.

If the affected bone is not a weight bearing one, the consequences are minimal. Children aged 10–15 are particularly prone to develop transient inflammation of the tuberosity of the tibia and the patella. These resolve satisfactorily with symptomatic treatment.

Further reading

Sharrard W.J. (1971) *Paediatric Orthopaedics and Fractures*. Blackwell Scientific Publications, Oxford.

McKusick V.A. (1972) *Heritable Disorders of Connective Tissue*. C. V. Mosby. Saint Louis.

Chapter 14

THE COLLAGEN DISEASES

Rheumatic fever and chorea are primarily conditions of childhood. Rheumatoid arthritis, systemic lupus and polyarteritis nodosa are primarily diseases of adults. Henoch–Schönlein syndrome is an important childhood condition and is grouped with the other collagen diseases because of some similarities to them.

RHEUMATIC FEVER (acute rheumatism)

Rheumatic fever is still the most important cause of acquired heart disease in children, but it is becoming less common and less severe.

Aetiology

It occurs mainly between the ages of 5–15 years. It is common in poor socio-economic conditions and there is a slight familial tendency. It appears to result from a hypersensitivity reaction to a beta haemolytic streptococcal infection. Typically this has been in the form of an acute tonsillitis 1–5 weeks previously.

Features

The major features are:
1   Polyarthritis. Medium sized joints are affected—the knees, elbows and ankles. Pain tends to 'flit' from joint to joint as the arthritis affects one joint for a day or two, subsides, and then affects another joint.

2   Skin rashes. The only pathognomonic rash is erythema marginatum, a serpiginous red rash with a raised edge which is most often found on the trunk. It occurs in about 10% of patients. Other non-specific rashes are common, and erythema nodosum may occur.

3   Carditis. Tachycardia and a short systolic murmur are invariably present. More certain evidence of cardiac involvement is a pansystolic or diastolic murmur, a pericardial friction rub or cardiac enlargement. Prolongation of the P-R interval is an early ECG change. Cardiac failure may occur.

4   Rheumatic nodules. These are found subcutaneously over bony prominences such as the shins, ulnar border of the forearms, the back of the hand, the spine and the occiput. They are no bigger than a pea and are not tender. It is unusual to find them except in severe and well established disease.

5   Chorea. (Sydenham's chorea, St. Vitus's dance). These involuntary movements are uncommon but may occur in older children late in the illness. Characteristically, there are involuntary, movements weakness and poor coordination of voluntary movement. Sometimes, particularly in girls, chorea appears as an isolated finding without other features of rheumatic fever.

Of these 5 major diagnostic features, any or all may be present. In addition there are important non-specific features: the child may be feverish and feel ill. Abdominal pain, chest pain, and nose bleeds may occur.

Investigations

The blood shows a normal white cell count or a neutrophil leukocytosis; mild hypochromic anaemia is common. The ESR and C-reactive protein levels are very high. Serial antistreptolysin O (ASO) titres show a sustained rise.

Management

Bed rest is usually imposed for a month followed by a further month of convalescence. If heart involvement is pronounced the duration of rest is increased.

Salicylates are essential and relieve the symptoms dramatically. They are given in large doses, e.g. 120 mg/kg/day, though the dose sometimes has to be reduced if tinnitus, tachypnoea or other signs of aspirin toxicity occur. Corticosteroids may be used if there is carditis.

A course of penicillin is given to eradicate any streptococcus, and is followed by prolonged prophylaxis. Anyone who has had rheumatic fever is at risk of a recurrence; daily oral penicillin reduces the chance of recurrence, and should be continued throughout childhood and adolescence.

Outcome

Carditis may cause permanent damage. The mitral and aortic valves are most frequently damaged, mitral stenosis being the commonest long-term complication. Permanent heart damage is commoner in the younger child; most older children with rheumatic fever do not have serious cardiac involvement. There are never any joint sequelae, the original lesion being a poly-synovitis rather than a true arthritis.

RHEUMATOID ARTHRITIS

Under the age of 7 it presents in a characteristic way that may be called 'Still's disease'. Systemic features predominate: there is fever, splenomegaly, lymphadenopathy and transient rashes. Joint involvement may be comparatively mild. Although there is a raised ESR and white cell count, serum latex and Rose-Waaler tests are usually negative.

Over the age of 7 the adult pattern of illness is seen with joint involvement and little or no systemic upset. The main feature of rheumatoid arthritis is the symmetrical involvement of both medium-sized joints and the small joints of the fingers, neck and temporo-mandibular joint (temporo-mandibular arthritis is pathognomonic of rheumatoid arthritis).

50% of children make a complete recovery, but the rest run a chronic relapsing course. Salicylates and physiotherapy are the mainstay of treatment.

SYSTEMIC LUPUS ERYTHEMATOSUS (SLE) AND POLYARTERITIS NODOSA (PAN)

The other collagen diseases are rare in children and extremely rare under the age of 8. SLE is the least rare, tending to occur in girls. Its manifestations are as varied as in adults though hepato-splenomegaly is a more constant finding. The most serious aspect is renal involvement which may lead to renal failure. Steroids are helpful but whether they affect the ultimate poor prognosis is uncertain.

HENOCH–SCHÖNLEIN SYNDROME
(Anaphylactoid Purpura, Allergic Purpura)

The syndrome is commonest in children aged 2–10 and is composed of four groups of symptoms: skin, joint, alimentary tract, and renal.

Skin

The rash is distributed over extensor surfaces of the limbs, particularly about the ankles and on the buttocks (Fig. 37). It

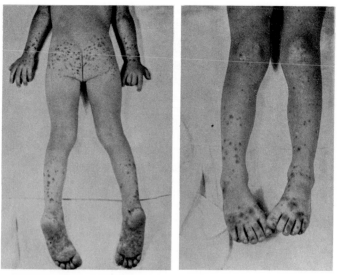

Fig. 37. Henoch–Schönlein purpura. The rash is symmetrically distributed and is most marked on the ankles, buttocks and extensor surfaces.

begins as a maculo-papular red rash, or as an urticarial rash in children under the age of 5, which gradually becomes purpuric. (The platelet count is normal or mildly decreased.) Swelling of the face, hands and feet is common and subcutaneous bleeds may occur in the scrotum, eyelids and conjunctiva.

Joints

Pain (arthralgia) of medium-sized joints is common and may progress to an obvious arthritis with red, swollen, tender joints.

Alimentary system

Colicky abdominal pain occurs and may be severe enough to mimic an acute abdominal emergency. Vomiting and diarrhoea are common; haematemesis and melaena less common, and intussusception or perforation very rare.

Renal

Haematuria is common, and in some cases the glomerulonephritis causes an acute nephritic syndrome, a nephrotic syndrome or renal insufficiency. The renal complications are responsible for the main morbidity and mortality of Henoch–Schönlein syndrome.

The four groups of symptoms generally present within a week of each other, but may occur in any order and persist for several weeks. Recurrence of any symptoms may occur for up to 6 months after onset. The cause is unknown and treatment is symptomatic.

Further reading

Sutton M.G.S. & Rubenstein D. (1974) Rheumatic fever. *British Journal of Hospital Medicine*, **12**, 691.

Schlesinger B.E., Forsyth C.C., White R.H.R., Smellie J.M. & Stroud C.E. (1961) Still's disease. *Archives of Disease in Childhood*, **36**, 65.

Meadow S.R., Glasgow E.W., White R.H.R., Moncrieff M.W., Cameron J.S. & Ogg C.S. (1972) Schonlein–Henoch syndrome. *Quarterly Journal of Medicine*, **41**, 243.

Chapter 15

THE SKIN

Skin disorders are a common reason for children being taken to the doctor. The infant's skin with its thin epidermis and immature glands is particularly liable to infection and blistering. Birthmarks, infections, eczema and napkin rashes are common. Fortunately the child's skin is capable of rapid healing, and is not usually affected by some of the more chronic adult conditions such as psoriasis.

BIRTHMARKS

Birthmarks may be the result of (a) developmental anomalies of the blood vessels—haemangiomas, or (b) an excess of pigment in the skin.

(a) The main types of haemangioma are:

Stork mark (Fig. 38)

This is a flat pinkish capillary haemangioma at the nape of the neck and also between the eyebrows of the infant (as if the stork had pecked the baby with its beak). They appear more red when the baby cries, but fade gradually during the first 2 years.

Strawberry naevus (Fig. 39)

This is a soft raised bright red capillary haemangioma often containing or overlying a more bluish cavernous haemangioma. It is not apparent until a few days after birth, and usually enlarges during the first 6 months. Thereafter sunken whitish areas develop in the lump and it gradually becomes paler and flatter. Most have disappeared by the age of 7 years, so that surgery or other treatment is best reserved for the very few which are extremely unsightly, do not regress spontaneously, or are expanding rapidly. In general spontaneous regression does not leave a noticeable scar, whilst treatment often does.

Port wine stain

Port wine stain is a capillary haemangioma which forms a flat dark purple patch of skin which looks ugly. It does not fade.

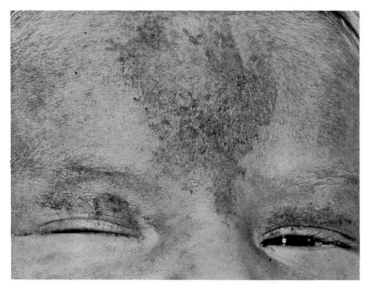

Fig. 38. Stork mark. This capillary haemangioma characteristically lies just above the nose. The upper eyelids are quite commonly affected, as in this baby.

Treatment is difficult, and camouflage with cosmetics is often the best treatment. *Sturge-Weber syndrome* is a rare association of a unilateral port wine stain of the face (usually involving the areas supplied by the 1st or 2nd divisions of the trigeminal nerve) and an intracranial haemangioma of the pia-arachnoid on the same side. Affected children may present with fits or neurological signs.

(b) Small **pigmented birthmarks** (pigmented moles) usually develop after the age of 2. They are common and rarely cause anxiety to parents.

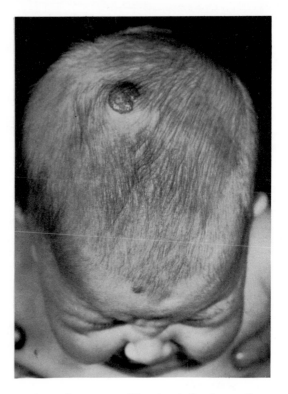

Fig. 39. A strawberry naevus. There is a similar, but smaller, naevus on the forehead.

Mongolian blue spots

These are large blue grey areas most common over the sacrum and buttocks, which look rather like bruises. They are only found in infants of Oriental or Negro stock, and gradually fade so that they are rarely visible after the age of 5.

RASHES

Napkin rash (Ammoniacal dermatitis)

This erythematous rash is common in infants and is found on the convexities of the buttocks, inner thighs, and genitalia (Fig. 40a). Fresh urine does not injure the skin, but prolonged contact with

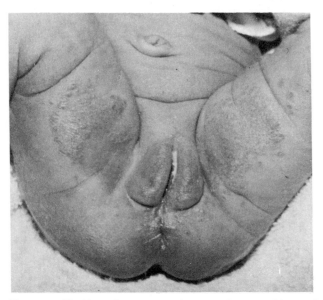

Fig. 40a. Napkin rash—most prominent on the convexities, and sparing skin creases.

stale urine which has broken down to form ammonia products does. The skin creases, which do not come into contact with the sodden nappy, are spared. In severe cases (Fig. 40b) papules and vesicles form which ulcerate leaving a moist surface which easily becomes secondarily infected either with pyogenic organisms or monilia (Fig. 40c). Secondary infection with monilia usually does involve the skin creases; it causes oval macules, vesicles, and a raised pimply margin to the rash.

It is impossible for mothers to change their baby's nappy immediately it is wet. Nappy rashes occur in all classes of society and are not simply confined to babies who have poor care. Some babies have a more sensitive skin than others, and are prone to

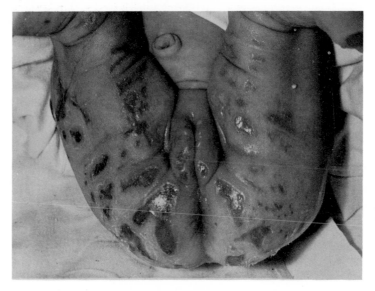

Fig. 40b. Severe napkin rash with secondary ulceration.

develop the rash. This must be explained to the mother to dispel needless guilt. However, gross ulcerated and chronic napkin rashes are a sign of inadequate care.

Treatment is based on the mother carrying out as many of the following instructions as are practicable: frequent and prompt changing of wet nappies including washing and drying the baby's perineum carefully; thorough washing of the nappies using a final rinse in an antiseptic such as cetrimide; rubbing a barrier cream or benzalkonium cream on the napkin area; avoiding plastic pants until the rash is cured as these create a hot steamy environment inside; using a 'nappy liner'—a thin specially treated piece of material which transmits moisture to the nappy but remains dry itself. In severe cases the most effective treatment is exposure of the moist rash in a warm dry environment, leaving the nappies off for a few days, together with the use of hydrocortisone cream to suppress the inflammation. Secondary infection requires local bactericidal or fungicidal cream.

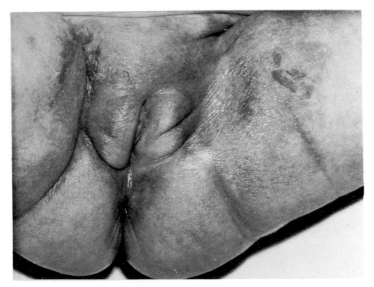

Fig. 40c. Napkin rash secondarily infected with monilia (which involves the skin creases).

Seborrhoeic dermatitis

Dandruff and scurf are the commonest manifestations in older children; but in infants *Cradle Cap* is common. This is a thick light brown crust over the top of the scalp, which may look quite difficult to remove. Most chemists sell proprietary brands of 'cradle cap remover' shampoo with which to wash the baby's scalp; alternatively salicylic acid and sulphur cream may be rubbed in before washing the hair. Regular washing of the scalp with soap or shampoo helps to prevent recurrence.

Eczema

This is common in atopic children whose families give a history of asthma, eczema or hay fever. The child is also at risk for asthma or hay fever. The erythematous scaling rash usually appears before the age of 6 months, and in infants usually involves the face, scalp and trunk (infantile eczema—Fig. 41). There is

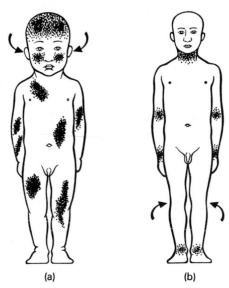

Fig. 41. Distribution of eczema.
(a) infancy: cheeks, scalp and behind ears are commonly affected.
(b) later childhood: skin flexures particularly antecubital and popliteal fossae.

intense itching, and scratching frequently leads to secondary infection (Fig. 42). The condition fluctuates, resolves completely in some children but in others persists in a mild form or periodically recurs. After infancy the rash is characteristically distributed in the skin flexures, particularly in the antecubital and popliteal fossae (flexural eczema—Fig. 41). Prolonged inflammation leads to thick lichenified skin and local lymph gland enlargement.

Frequent bathing in a bath to which emulsifying ointment has been added is followed by the local application of steroids.

Bactericidal creams are used for secondary infection. Antihist-amines, particularly trimeprazine, subdue the itching. Other measures may include hypnotics at night, and restraining clothing such as cloth mittens which are then fastened to the cot side to

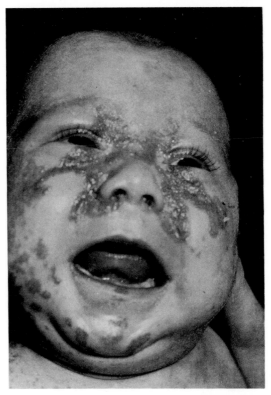

Fig. 42. Infantile eczema involving the face and leading to secondary bacterial infection.

prevent the infant scratching. The condition tends to improve, and certainly becomes more manageable as the child becomes older.

Impetigo

This is a skin infection caused by staphylococci or sometimes streptococci. It commonly involves the face, around the mouth and nose, and also the hands. It begins as a small red spot which rapidly ulcerates, producing exudate which dries in a golden brown crust over the red itching skin beneath. Spread may be rapid and the child scratching the lesion may spread it to other parts of the body or to other members of the family. It is very contagious, therefore the child should be excluded from school until it is healed. Impetigo frequently complicates infestation with scabies or pediculosis (see below).

Treatment involves bathing the lesions in cetrimide and water to remove the crusts and then applying an antibiotic cream such as tetracycline. Systemic antibiotics may be added if the child is febrile or the rash severe. The family must be warned about the risk of becoming infected themselves and the affected child should use a separate towel and face cloth.

Urticaria (Hives)

Urticaria is common in children, especially under the age of 5. It is characterized by red blotches and whitish wheals which itch. They disappear and reappear over a period of hours or days. Sometimes sensitivity to a particular drug or food appears to be responsible. Treatment is symptomatic; systemic antihistamines or adrenaline may produce dramatic relief. *Papular Urticaria* consists of hard papules most often on the limbs. They appear in crops and itch so that secondary infection is common. In many children they are associated with insect bites, fleas, lice and bed bugs.

Erythema nodosum

The tender shiny red lumps are 1–3 cms in diameter. They are most commonly distributed symmetrically over the front of the shins, but do occur elsewhere. During the first week they become more protuberant, purple and painful, then during the next 2 weeks gradually subside and look like old bruises. They may occur at intervals in crops. Although they are thought to represent a hypersensitivity phenomenon to certain stimuli, the provocative stimulus frequently cannot be identified. In childhood the important associations are:

1 Streptococcal infection;
2 Tuberculosis;
3 Certain drugs;
4 Rare childhood diseases such as sarcoidosis, lupus erythematosus and ulcerative colitis.

INFESTATIONS

Pediculosis

The commonest louse infestation in childhood is with the head louse (*pediculosis capitis*). The louse lives in the hair and lives off blood which it gets by biting the scalp. It causes irritation, and the combination of the bites and the child scratching frequently leads to impetigo and enlarged occipital and cervical lymph glands. The bites may resemble purpura confined to the neck and shoulders. Sometimes the lice can be seen, but more often just the tiny whitish eggs (nits) are seen attached singly to the hair. They can be identified with certainty beneath a microscope; they are ovoid with one blunt end and one pointed end by which they are stuck to the hair shaft. Applications of dicophane (DDT) or gamma benzene hexachloride are rubbed into the hair and left for 24 hours before it is washed. Other members of the home should be examined for similar infestation.

Scabies

The mite *Sarcoptes scabiei* lays its eggs in burrows beneath the skin. The larva migrates and burrows into the skin, gradually developing into the adult mite, which re-emerges, becomes impregnated and burrows to lay more eggs. After a few weeks the child becomes sensitized and develops a very itchy papulovesicular rash. In older children this is most marked in the interdigital spaces, wrist flexures and anterior axillary folds. In infants it frequently involves the face, trunk and feet. The burrows can be seen as small linear elevations of skin adjacent to a small vesicle, but they are often obscured by excoriation and secondary infection. Diagnosis is confirmed by microscopic identification of a mite from one of the burrows. Scabies has become increasingly common in Britain and should be considered as a possible cause for any unexplained itching rash. The infestation is transferred by bodily contact, so that other members of the family are usually affected, and all those living together should be treated at the same time. After a hot bath and much scrubbing, 25% benzyl benzoate emulsion is painted over all the body except the head. The application is repeated on the second and third days followed by another hot bath on the fourth day. Disinfestation of clothing and bedding is advised.

Further reading

Forfar J.O. & Arneil G.C. (eds) (1973) Diseases of the skin. Chapter 24, *Textbook of Paediatrics*. Churchill Livingstone, Edinburgh and London.

Chapter 16

THE URINARY TRACT

DEVELOPMENT

The fetus excretes urine from the 12th week of intra-uterine life, and by term it is both swallowing and excreting 500 ml/day. This function is more important for the production of amniotic fluid than for elimination of waste products, since the fetus is being effectively haemodialysed by the placenta.

At birth renal function is limited. The baby can cope well with normal food intake simply because body growth is rapid and milk contains exactly the right substances required for growth with very little excess. When this situation is altered the limitations of the immature kidney are seen. If the neonate has a small excess of intravenous fluid it becomes oedematous. If it has diarrhoea the kidneys fail to conserve fluid adequately. Compared with the adult a relatively small decrease in renal perfusion, e.g. from mild dehydration or cardiac failure, may result in a raised blood urea level.

Although glomerular function is limited during the first year it is relatively more efficient than tubular function. Morphologically the glomeruli, which are half adult size at birth, are relatively larger than the tubules. As the kidney matures tubular growth and function increase faster so that by the age of 1 year the adult pattern of function is present. Renal growth continues throughout childhood by means of increase in nephron size, and not by the production of new nephrons. A steady increase of size of renal outline, as seen on X-ray, is a useful sign of healthy growing kidneys.

URINE EXAMINATION

pH

A pH of 5 or 6 is usual. Alkaline urine is more likely in infants than in older children because of the frequent feeds. It also occurs after alkaline medicines; sometimes in the presence of urine infection, and as a result of very rare tubular abnormalities.

Albumin

20% of children have a trace of albumin in their urine; it can be disregarded. 5% have 0.3 g/l or more. If this is persistent a 24-hour collection is made; an excretion of over 0.3 g/day requires further investigation. Transient albuminuria may occur with fever or hard exercise. Postural (orthostatic) proteinuria is commonest in the 10–15-year-old age group.

Glucose

Glycosuria is rare. Likely causes are a low renal threshold or diabetes mellitus.

Ketones

Ketonuria is common, particularly in ill children who are anorexic or have been vomiting.

Formed elements

Careful collection of the specimen is vital. In infants this may have to be by means of a self-adhesive perineal bag, which must be emptied immediately urine has been passed in order to avoid perineal contamination.

White blood cells (pus cells)

A healthy boy may have up to 5 WBC/mm³ and a girl up to 50/mm³. An excess of white cells is commonly the result of vulval contamination in girls. In a carefully collected or mid-stream specimen it may be the result of a urine infection or an abnormality of the renal tract (Fig. 43).

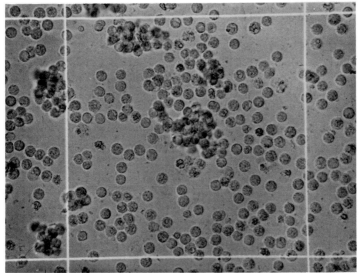

Fig. 43. Gross pyuria. The urine contained more than 40,000 WBC/mm³, many of them aggregated in clumps. The granular appearance of nucleated white cells is visible on either low or high power microscopy.

Red blood cells (RBC)

They may be difficult to identify in urine, but any significant number is likely to be associated with a positive dip stick chemical test for haemoglobin. Urine should not contain more than 2 RBC/mm³. The commonest causes of haematuria are glomerulonephritis and urinary tract infection. Casts should be searched for to localize the site of the blood loss.

Casts

Casts are formed in the renal tubules. Cellular casts may be composed of renal tubular cells but more commonly are composed of red cells, or disintegrating red cells (granular casts). They are an important sign of glomerulonephritis. Hyaline casts devoid of cells are invariably present whenever there is proteinuria, and a few may be present in a concentrated early morning specimen from a normal child.

Bacteria

If the urine is infected bacteria can usually be seen as motile rods, even in unspun unstained urine using the low power objective. They can be identified more certainly under high power (Fig. 44).

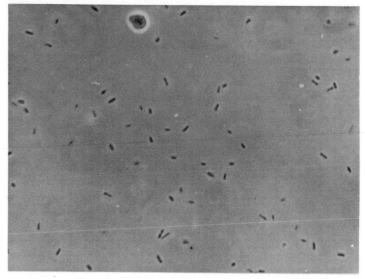

Fig. 44. Bacteriuria. Infected urine viewed under high power; many of the organisms were motile. There is a white cell at the top of the picture.

CONGENITAL ANOMALIES

Agenesis

This is the result of the ureteric bud failing to develop so that the ureter and kidney are absent. If unilateral the child may live a full and healthy life provided the other kidney is normal. Bilateral agenesis is lethal. Oligohydramnios has usually been noted during pregnancy, and a proportion of affected infants have a characteristic facial appearance (Potter's syndrome).

Hypoplastic kidneys

These are deficient in renal parenchyma. They are not usually associated with other abnormalities.

Dysplastic kidneys

These contain abnormally differentiated parenchyma. They are commonly associated with obstruction and other abnormalities of the urinary tract. *Cystic disease* represents one form of renal dysplasia. Infantile polycystic disease is associated with massive kidneys, renal failure early in life and a recessive pattern of inheritance, whereas adult polycystic disease which has a dominant inheritance is generally not detected in early life because the kidneys are not enlarged and function well during childhood.

Ureteric abnormalities

Obstruction

This is commonest at the pelvi-ureteric junction where it may cause hydronephrosis and permanent renal damage. *Duplication* of the ureter and pelvis may occur on one or both sides. If it only affects the upper half of the ureter it is not important, but if it extends down to the bladder so that there are two separate ureteric openings on that side there are commonly obstructions or abnormalities of the lower ureter. A *ureterocele* is a cystic enlargement of the ureter within the bladder which may cause obstruction.

Bladder and urethral abnormalities

Posterior urethral valves

These are an important cause of obstruction to urine flow and occur almost exclusively in boys. Bladder neck obstruction is more rare. They usually present in the newborn period or at least in the first year as acute obstruction or chronic partial obstruction with dribbling micturition.

N.B. Obstruction of the lower urinary tract is frequently associated with renal dysplasia. But regardless of potential renal function, obstruction may cause direct damage by back pressure or predispose to urinary tract infection which may cause further damage. Most obstructive abnormalities can be corrected by surgery.

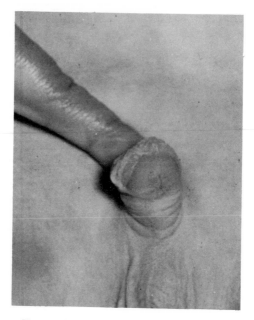

Fig. 45. Hypospadias. The meatus is at the junction of the glans and shaft. The prepuce is characteristically misshapen and hooded.

Hypospadias

The urethral opening is on the ventral surface of the penis (Fig. 45). If it is at the junction of the glans and shaft no treatment is needed, but if it is on the shaft of the penis plastic surgery is required before school entry. The foreskin may be needed for this reconstruction, therefore boys with hypospadias should not be circumcized.

RENAL DISEASE

TERMINOLOGY AND CLASSIFICATION

In recent years nephrologists have begun to use the same language as each other. This is a major advance, and the starting point for understanding renal disease is to appreciate the classifications that are used.

Firstly, syndromes—collections of symptoms and signs, are defined, e.g. nephrotic syndrome or acute nephritic syndrome.

Secondly, a pathological or morphological description is given. This is obtained from biopsy or autopsy, e.g. proliferative glomerulonephritis or 'minimal changes'.

Thirdly, an aetiological label is added when this is known, e.g. 'diabetic' or 'post-streptococcal'.

Whilst there are certain correlations between these three levels of diagnosis, it is essential to realize that a particular morphological appearance (for instance, proliferative glomerulonephritis) may be found in each of several different clinical syndromes. Further, a syndrome may be associated with several different morphological pictures, and have a variety of different aetiologies.

The most important syndromes of renal disease in childhood are:—

Acute nephritic syndrome;
Recurrent haematuria;
Nephrotic syndrome;
Symptomless proteinuria;
Urinary tract infection;
Renal failure.

ACUTE NEPHRITIC SYNDROME

This is characterized by haematuria, oliguria, hypertension and a raised blood urea. The last two features are not always present.

Aetiology

The best-known form is post-streptococcal glomerulonephritis, sometimes called acute nephritis (Ellis type I nephritis). The child has had a beta-haemolytic streptococcal infection, usually a pharyngitis, 1–2 weeks previously. Immune complexes composed of streptococci, antibody and complement are deposited in the glomeruli. There they provoke proliferation of the endothelial cells (proliferative glomerulonephritis). Post-streptococcal glomerulonephritis which was once a common condition is now uncommon in Britain.

An acute nephritic syndrome may also occur at the time of pneumococcal pneumonia, septicaemia and some viral infections. It is sometimes seen in Henoch–Schönlein syndrome and the collagen diseases.

Features

Acute nephritic syndrome has an age distribution with a peak at 7 years. The child is well until the sudden onset of illness and the appearance of bright red or brownish urine. Facial oedema, particularly of the eyelids, is common, and there may be abdominal or loin pain together with loin tenderness. The blood pressure is raised in half the children.

Investigations

A small volume of blood-stained urine is passed. In addition to copious red blood cells there is an excess of white cells and moderate proteinuria. Red cell and granular casts are present.

The blood urea is raised in two-thirds of children. Serial anti-streptolysin O (ASO) titres show a rise to above 1:250. Serum C_3 (B_1C) complement is reduced for 2–8 weeks after onset.

Course and Treatment

Oliguria lasts for only a few days. Diuresis usually occurs within a week and is accompanied by return of blood urea and blood pressure to normal. The haematuria and proteinuria gradually subside over the next year or so.

During the oliguric phase fluid and protein are restricted, but it is rarely necessary to start a strict renal failure regime. Penicillin is given for 3 months to reduce the chance of recurrence, which in any case is rare. Other treatment is symptomatic; the child is kept in bed only as long as he feels ill.

Over 80% make a full recovery, but a few develop progressive renal disease. Death in the acute phase from hypertensive encephalopathy, cardiac failure or acute renal failure is very rare.

RECURRENT HAEMATURIA SYNDROME

It is characterized by recurrent bouts of haematuria. These may occur at the time of a systemic infection or exertion. The child may feel mildly unwell but more often has no symptoms. The aetiology is uncertain.

Between attacks the urine is normal or shows microscopic haematuria. Proteinuria is less common and may indicate more serious renal disease.

Investigations are done to exclude other causes of haematuria: urine culture, IVP for a tumour or stone, and screening tests for bleeding disorders. If, as is usual, the urine contains red cell and granular casts cystoscopy constitutes an improper assault, since casts originate from the kidneys.

The prognosis is good. Renal function is normal and continues so in over 90%. The bouts of haematuria may continue for several years, and the doctor who has the task of reassuring the parents usually ends up wishing that blood was colourless. Prolonged restriction of activity or bed rest is more likely to result in an uneducated delinquent adolescent than to affect the renal prognosis.

NEPHROTIC SYNDROME

Nephrotic syndrome is characterized by heavy proteinuria, hypoalbuminaemia and oedema.

Features

It is commonest in boys aged 2–3 years. Apart from the gradual onset of generalized oedema the child may be well or only mildly off colour. Other symptoms are directly related to oedema, for instance discomfort from ascites or breathlessness from pleural effusion (Fig. 46).

Aetiology

Over 90% of childhood nephrotic syndrome is the result of primary renal disease of unknown cause. Nephrotic syndrome secondary to systemic illness is less common than in adults; the least rare causes being Henoch–Schönlein syndrome and the collagen diseases. In Africa, quartan malaria is an important cause.

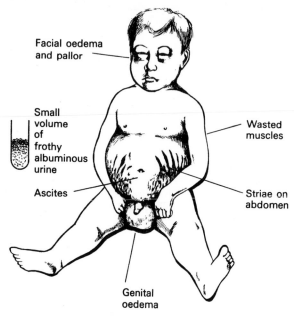

Facial oedema and pallor

Small volume of frothy albuminous urine

Ascites

Wasted muscles

Striae on abdomen

Genital oedema

Fig. 46. Nephrotic syndrome.

Pathology

Most kidneys show 'minimal changes' (formerly called lipoid nephrosis). This means that the biopsy appearance is normal or near normal on light microscopy.

Investigations

The urine is frothy and albuminous. The 24-hour excretion of protein is anything from 1–20 g. The protein excreted is mainly of small molecular weight, i.e. highly selective proteinuria. Hyaline casts are abundant. Serum albumin is below 25 g/l and the serum cholesterol is usually raised. Blood urea is normal.

Treatment and Prognosis

A high protein, low salt diet is given, and moderate fluid restriction imposed. Corticosteroids are given in large doses for 4–6 weeks. Diuretics may be needed if the oedema is causing symptoms. Most children go into remission within 10 days of starting steroids. Diuresis occurs and the oedema and albuminuria disappear rapidly. A large proportion relapse within the next year.

Table 11. Comparison of findings in acute nephritic syndrome, nephrotic syndrome and urinary tract infection

		Acute nephritic syndrome	Nephrotic syndrome	Urinary tract infection
Child	Oedema	Mild facial	Gross	0
	Blood pressure	Raised	Normal	Normal
Urine	Albumen	+ +	+ + + +	+ or 0
	RBC	+ + + +	0	+ or 0
	WBC	+ +	0	+/+ + +
	Casts	Cellular/granular	Hyaline	0
	Bacteria	0	0	+ + +

They can be given further courses of steroids, but if the relapses are frequent cyclophosphamide will usually produce a longer remission.

The long-term prognosis is better than it is for adults with nephrotic syndrome. Most children are well and have normal renal function 10 years later. A small proportion, including many of those initially unresponsive to steroids, develop renal insufficiency. Unusual features at onset which are unfavourable prognostic signs are: late age of onset, haematuria, hypertension, raised blood urea or urine containing a high proportion of large molecular weight proteins, i.e. poorly selective proteinuria. Renal biopsy tends to be reserved for children showing these features.

URINARY TRACT INFECTION

Infection of the urinary tract is one of the commonest and most puzzling conditions of childhood. Because it is unusual to be able to localize the infection to any particular site it is preferable to call it 'urinary tract infection' than to use words such as 'cystitis' or 'pyelitis'.

Incidence

From birth to adolescence the prevalence of urinary tract infection is just over 1%. In the neonatal period boys are more often infected: but thereafter girls predominate. By the age of 2 years, 5% of girls have had a urinary tract infection, and during the school years infection is 25 times more likely in a girl.

Pathology

The commonest pathogen is E. Coli. Bacteria of the same strain are usually present in the child's gut and it is assumed that the organism enters the urethra via the perineum.

Features

The child may have neither symptoms nor signs. When there are symptoms they tend to be non-specific: feeding problems, fever, prolonged jaundice in the neonate; vague malaise, enuresis or urgency in the older child. The classical adult picture of burning dysuria, fever and loin pain is uncommon in children.

Investigations

The diagnosis is made if a carefully collected clean specimen of urine contains more than 10^9 organisms/l in pure growth. A mixed growth is more likely to be the result of contamination than infection. A colony count of less than 10^8/l is normal, a count in between means that the culture must be repeated. Ideally a positive diagnosis should not be made unless 2 consecutive colony counts have contained more than 10^9 organisms/l. The greatest problem in infants is obtaining a clean urine sample. Occasionally it is necessary to resort to supra-pubic aspiration of urine directly from the bladder using a syringe and needle. The infant's bladder lies relatively high above the pubis so that it is not difficult to aspirate.

Macroscopically the urine may have an opalescent sheen. Microscopically bacteria are seen and leukocyturia is usual, boys having more than 5 WBC/mm^3 and girls more than 50 WBC/mm^3. The presence or absence of albuminuria is irrelevant to diagnosis. Microscopic haematuria may be present.

Management

1   Initial treatment. Appropriate chemotherapy is given for 10 days; sulphonamides are effective, safe and inexpensive. Fluid intake is increased and frequent micturition encouraged.

2   Further investigation. Ideally an intravenous pyelogram should be done on any child who has had a definite urinary infection. This should be followed by a micturating cystogram in most cases. The aim is to detect obstructive abnormalities. Renal stones are rare but other obstructive lesions are quite common. Vesico-ureteric reflux is found in a quarter of cases: as the bladder empties, urine refluxes up the ureter and then at the end of micturition falls back to form a stagnant residual pool (Fig. 48). Reflux is commoner in children than in adults, and providing recurrent infections can be prevented, for instance by prophylactic antibiotics, it tends to go as the child grows. If medical treatment is unsuccessful, surgical correction of the reflux is possible.

3   Follow up is the most important part of the management. One third of children will have a recurrence within the next year. It is as unrealistic to claim having 'cured' a urine infection on the basis of sterile urine two days after treatment as it would be to claim having 'cured' an asthmatic child on the basis of having stopped one bout of wheezing. The child's urine must be cultured a few days after completing the initial 10 days' therapy, and 1, 3, 6 and 12 months afterwards *even though the child is symptomless.*

The problem of prognosis

Infection of the renal parenchyma may cause permanent or progressive damage leading to renal insufficiency. The morphological description of such small scarred kidneys is chronic pyelonephritis. The same morphological appearance is seen in the final stages of progressive renal disease of many origins other than infection. It is clear that the vast majority of the multitude of children with urinary tract infection do not incur renal damage. Renal damage is most likely in those with recurrent infection and ureteric reflux under the age of 5. But this is a large

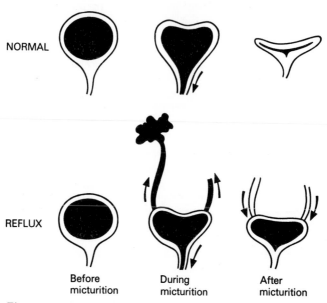

Fig. 47. Vesico-ureteric reflux. At the end of micturition there remains in the bladder a puddle of stagnant urine.

group of girls and most of them, even though they may have infections throughout childhood, have a fate no worse than 'honeymoon cystitis' and acute pyelitis of pregnancy.

We have no way of identifying the tiny minority whose kidneys are destined to be damaged by infection. Therefore as pyelonephritis may at present be the only preventable cause of renal failure an active policy has to be followed to detect, treat *and follow up* children with urinary tract infections.

RENAL FAILURE

Acute renal failure describes the situation in which previously healthy kidneys suddenly stop working. It is a rewarding condition to treat in childhood because a higher proportion of children have recoverable conditions than do adults who present acutely.

Progressive renal insufficiency or chronic renal failure is uncommon in children. During the early months of life congenital abnormalities, particularly renal dysplasia, are the main cause. Thereafter primary renal diseases (various forms of glomerulonephritis) are the commonest cause. Children with end-stage renal disease have the same features as adults, e.g. anaemia, hypertension and renal rickets; in addition they fail to grow. Facilities for regular dialysis and transplantation for children are available in most regions of Britain. At present a selective policy is being used; long-term maintenance therapy only being offered to certain children who have reached school age.

Further reading

Forfar J.O. & Arneil G.C. (1973) Disorders of the urogenital system. Chapter 17, *Textbook of Paediatrics*. Churchill Livingstone, Edinburgh and London.
Barnett H.L. & Einhorn A.H. (1972) The kidneys and urinary tract. Chapter 24, *Paediatrics*. Butterworths, London.
James J.A. (1972) *Renal Disease in Childhood*. C.V. Mosby, St Louis.
Williams D.I. (1974) *Paediatric Urology*. Butterworths, London.

Chapter 17

THE BLOOD

The normal blood picture

The neonate has a haemoglobin of 19 g/dl (130%). Erythropoiesis is limited during the early months, so that the haemoglobin level falls (Table 12). It reaches its lowest level of 11 g/dl (75%) at 3 months and thereafter rises steadily. These levels are normal at that age and therefore many people prefer to express children's haemoglobin levels as 'x g/dl' (or 'x g/100 ml') rather than as a percentage of the normal adult level. At birth haemoglobin is mainly of the fetal type—HbF. This combines more readily with oxygen at low oxygen tensions, and also gives up CO_2 more easily than does HbA, the adult type. During the first year HbF is gradually replaced by HbA. The white cell count is relatively higher throughout childhood, and in the early years there is a preponderance of lymphocytes which is particularly marked during the first year. Leukocytosis in response to infection is also more marked, and occasionally includes a few primitive white cells. In infants a lymphocytic response to infection does not exclude a bacterial cause. The platelet count is mildly reduced in the first few months but by 6 months the normal adult value of $250–350 \times 10^9/l$ is reached. The ESR should be below 16 in childhood, provided that the packed cell volume is at least 35%.

ANAEMIA

Anaemia is common in childhood, but not quite as common as many mothers suspect. Mothers are often worried by their child's pallor, which is more often a feature of a fair complexion than of anaemia. Anaemia may cause tiredness and even breathlessness,

Table 12. Normal blood picture

Age	Hb (g/dl)	Type	WBC × 10⁹/l	Lymphocytes
1–2 weeks	18	HbF > HbA	12.0	70%
1 month	14	HbF = HbA	11.0	65%
3 months	11	HbF < HbA	11.0	65%
1 year	12	HbA	10.0	55%
4 years	12	HbA	9.0	40%
12 years	14	HbA	8.0	30%

but most tired children are not anaemic. Examination of the mucous membranes will usually provide the most reliable information, followed if necessary by a blood test. It is imperative to report back to parents that a blood test is normal; many parents think a blood test is being done because the doctor suspects leukaemia.

Anaemia may be caused by:

1 Diminished production;
2 Excessive breakdown;
3 Blood loss.

1 Diminished production

A. Deficiency anaemias

Iron deficiency anaemia is by far the most common, and is characterized by a hypochromic microcytic blood picture (Fig. 48). The mean corpuscular haemoglobin concentration will be under 32 g/dl. Basically it is caused by insufficient intake of iron, but this is more likely for the following groups of children:

(i) Pre-term babies and twins (page 24)
(ii) Infants who have to exist entirely on milk and are late changing to iron-containing weaning foods—sometimes because the infant is retarded or has cerebral palsy and is late learning to chew solids
(iii) Children from poor homes who have inadequate diets and little meat, or who suffer from chronic or recurrent infections which suppress appetite and depress bone marrow haemopoiesis.

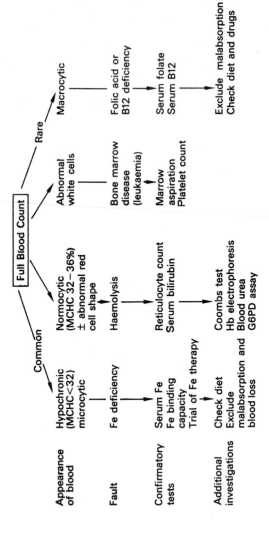

Fig. 48. The investigation of anaemia.

(iv) Children with malabsorption who fail to absorb the iron in their diet.

(v) Adolescent girls who are undergoing a phase of rapid growth at a time when they are also losing blood from menstruation.

Treatment is aimed at identifying the causes of the deficiency and correcting them. Oral iron preparations provoke a rapid reticulocytosis in most cases. Oral iron should be given prophylactically to those children most at risk for iron deficiency anaemia—pre-term and twin babies up to the age of 6 months, and children having inadequate diets.

Other deficiency anaemias are uncommon. Folic acid deficiency in British children may be seen in malabsorption syndromes; it rarely results from dietary deficiency. Pernicious anaemia is extremely rare in children. Hypothyroidism and scurvy are associated with hypochromic anaemias which are corrected by treatment of the primary condition.

B. Bone marrow disturbance

Infiltration. Leukaemia (page 206) is the most important infiltrative disturbance which may present as anaemia. Secondary deposits from malignant tumours and lipidoses are less common.

Toxic Damage. Chronic infection and renal insufficiency depress haemopoiesis. A large number of poisons may suppress the cellular elements of the marrow and cause an *aplastic anaemia*. These include drugs such as chloramphenicol and troxidone.

2 Excessive breakdown

Haemolytic anaemias are not as common as deficiency anaemias, but are important in childhood as some are specific to children and others cause their main problems in childhood. They are characterized by chronic or recurrent normochromic anaemia. While haemolysis is active there is usually a reticulocytosis, but there is sometimes marrow aplasia at the time of acute haemolysis. When the haemolysis is severe and sudden it is called a 'haemolytic crisis'; jaundice, dark urine and dark stools are likely. Splenomegaly is a feature of chronic cases.

The main cause for the haemolysis may be an abnormality of the red blood cell, or an abnormal factor in the circulation.

A. Cellular abnormalities

These can be conveniently grouped according to the way in which the abnormality is identified either by red cell shape, enzyme abnormality, or abnormal haemoglobin.

(i) Red cell shape. The most important abnormality is *Hereditary Spherocytosis* (acholuric jaundice) in which the red cells are fragile spherocytes and haemolyse easily. It is inherited as a dominant characteristic, but one-third of those affected have a negative family history.

(ii) Enzyme defect. The commonest defect is *Glucose-6-phosphate dehydrogenase (G6PD) deficiency* which occurs in Britain but which is more common in those of Mediterranean or African origin and may be inherited as a sex-linked recessive condition. Affected children are susceptible to certain chemicals which cause haemolysis in them but not in normal people. The list of possible chemicals is long but most children with G6PD deficiency are harmed by only a few of them. PAS, primaquine and aniline derivatives are particularly frequent pathogenic agents. Some of the children develop haemolysis after eating the bean or inhaling the pollen of the Fava bean (a type of broad bean); this is called favism.

(iii) *Haemoglobinopathies.* Many different types of abnormal haemoglobin have been described, but there are only two important diseases caused by the abnormality: Thalassaemia and sickle cell disease. Children with *thalassaemia* have a persistent preponderance of HbF and a deficiency of HbA. It is most common in those of Mediterranean stock, and is inherited by autosomal recessive genes. Those with the heterozygous state have thalassaemia minor, and are asymptomatic or have a mild anaemia. Their red cells contain up to 20% HbF. Those with the homozygous state, thalassaemia major (Cooley's anaemia) develop severe haemolysis and anaemia in infancy. The children grow poorly and develop massive hepatosplenomegaly. Hyperplasia of the bone marrow leads to thickened skull bones. Blood transfusions correct the anaemia temporarily, but survival into adulthood is unusual.

Sickle cell disease occurs in the negro races. HbS is present in place of HbA. At low oxygen tensions the cell becomes crescent or sickle shaped and is likely to haemolyse. The heterozygotes have about 30% HbS, may show sickling, but are usually symptomless. The homozygotes develop recurrent episodes of haemolysis during infancy. In addition to the problems of haemolytic and aplastic episodes which occur in any haemolytic anaemia, those with sickle cell disease also may develop intravascular thromboses. The thrombotic episodes cause local pain in the abdomen, bones and joints. The abdominal pain is commonly severe with signs resembling an acute abdominal emergency together with fever and leukocytosis. Treatment is symptomatic, and the prognosis poor; many die in late childhood or early adult life from infections, cardiac failure, or thrombotic episodes.

B. Extracellular abnormalities

Antibodies causing premature destruction of the red cell are usually associated with a positive Coombs' test. Apart from haemolytic disease of the newborn (page 27) circulating factors causing haemolysis are not common in childhood.

Haemolytic anaemia may occur secondary to malignancy or lupus erythematosus (rare in childhood) or as a complication of severe poisoning or infection.

3 Blood Loss

Hidden blood loss is not common in childhood, peptic ulcers and gastrointestinal malignancy being very rare. Gastrointestinal bleeding from a Meckel's diverticulum or a hiatus hernia is more likely to present with overt bleeding than unexplained anaemia.

COAGULATION DISORDERS

Haemophilia

Most cases (Haemophilia A) are caused by deficiency of plasma factor VIII. A minority are caused by deficiency of factor IX (Christmas disease or Haemophilia B). Both are caused by sex linked recessive genes, so that half the sons of the asymptomatic female carriers are affected. The condition usually presents during the second or third year of life, with bleeding following a trivial injury. Bleeding into soft tissues or into joints is particularly common. The haemarthroses particularly involving the knees are one of the major problems of haemophilia; recurrent haemarthrosis leads to permanent joint damage and chronic disability. The blood shows a prolonged clotting time and partial thromboplastin time (PTT); specific assay of the relevant coagulation factors is then performed to identify the precise abnormality. Treatment aims at raising the level of the relevant coagulation factor as rapidly as possible to stop bleeding, and replacing blood loss if necessary. Usually a transfusion of fresh frozen plasma or an injection of a plasma concentrate (e.g. cryoprecipitate) is sufficient. Haemarthroses require careful orthopaedic management. One of the most difficult problems is in protecting the child from trauma by special schooling and forbidding certain activities, and yet allowing the child to lead an enjoyable and profitable life. Regular prophylactic dental care is important. The condition usually becomes less severe as adult life is reached. Regional centres are being set up to provide skilled coordinated care for haemophiliacs.

Thrombocytopaenia

Thrombocytopaenia may be a feature of several systemic diseases as well as infiltrative diseases of the bone marrow and marrow aplasia.

However the most common thrombocytopaenic purpura of childhood is *Idiopathic Thrombocytopaenic Purpura (ITP)*, which occurs in healthy school children and is associated with a normal or near normal bone marrow which contains an excess of immature megakaryocytes. The onset is acute, often occurring 1–3 weeks after an upper respiratory tract infection. A widespread petechial rash appears, developing into small purpuric spots. Purpuric spots do not fade when pressed; other causes of purpura are shown in Table 13. There may be bleeding from the nose or into the mucous membranes. Apart from the signs of bleeding there are no other abnormal signs, and the haemoglobin and white cell count are normal. The platelet count is low, usually below 30×10^9/l. During the onset period severe bleeding may occur, but generally the outcome is good. 75% of children have

Table 13. The main causes of purpura in childhood

Platelet count low (thrombocytopaenia)	Platelet count normal
Idiopathic thrombocytopaenic purpura	Henoch–Schönlein syndrome
Leukaemia (page 206)	Septicaemia (particularly meningococcal)
Toxic effect of drugs	Common infectious illnesses and viraemia
	Uraemia

made a complete recovery within one month of onset and have no further trouble. Transfusions of platelets and blood may be needed at onset. Corticosteroids, given in large doses, reduce the risk of massive haemorrhage and accelerate the natural recovery in most children. Splenectomy is reserved for the small minority who have persistent or recurrent thrombocytopaenia.

Disseminated Intravascular Coagulation (DIC, consumption coagulopathy, fibrinolysis)

This syndrome is becoming increasingly recognized as an important cause of bleeding and purpura. It is convenient (though an oversimplification) to consider that intravascular coagulation uses up platelets and other factors, causing overt bleeding elsewhere; and that as the circulating blood is forced through the intravascular clots some of the red cells are damaged, become fragmented and haemolyse. Therefore, the syndrome is associated with bleeding and a haemolytic anaemia, and may be diagnosed by the presence of fragmented red cells, thrombocytopaenia and deficiency of coagulation factors. In the neonate it occurs as a result of severe anoxia or massive infection. In older children it may be associated with septicaemia, cyanotic congenital heart disease and vasculitis.

Further reading

Hardisty R.M. & Weatherall D.G. (1974) *Blood and its Disorders.* Blackwell Scientific Publications, Oxford.

Smith C.H. (1966) *Blood Diseases of Infancy and Childhood.* C.V. Mosby, St. Louis.

Mauer A.M. (1973) *Paediatric Haematology.* McGraw Hill.

Chapter 18

MALIGNANT DISEASE

Malignant disease is the second most frequent cause of death between the ages of 1 and 15 years. Accidents are the commonest cause of death. Although malignancy is an important cause of death, it is nevertheless uncommon—a general practitioner can expect to see one child with malignant disease every 20 years.

Malignancy is not only less common than in adults, it is also different in origin and course. The classical epithelial malignancies of adult life, carcinomata of the respiratory, gastrointestinal and reproductive tracts, are rarely seen in childhood. Most childhood malignancy arises from the reticuloendothelial system or from nerve or connective tissue. Primitive tumours, blast cell tumours and sarcomata are relatively more common. Childhood tumours are relatively more malignant, disseminating early and responding poorly to treatment.

RETICULOENDOTHELIAL TUMOURS

These are the commonest childhood malignancy. Three quarters can be classified as leukaemia, a quarter are non-leukaemic tumours.

Leukaemia

This is nearly always acute lymphoblastic in type. It is commoner in boys and the peak age of onset is from 2–5 years. The presentation is likely to result from anaemia causing pallor and lethargy, or from thrombocytopaenia causing purpura and bleeding. Fever is common, and leukaemic deposits in the bones may cause limb pain. Lymphadenopathy, hepatomegaly and splenomegaly are variable, and frequently not present at onset.

Diagnosis is usually possible from examination of the peripheral blood; anaemia and thrombocytopaenia are associated with lymphoblast cells. The total white cell count is more often normal or decreased ('aleukaemic' leukaemia) than raised at onset. Later on leukocytosis may be seen. The diagnosis is confirmed by bone marrow examination.

Treatment consists of corticosteroids and cytotoxic drugs combined with supportive therapy in the form of blood or platelet transfusions and antibiotics.

80% of children will achieve a remission within one month and be active and happy by then. Subsequent relapse will occur and can be treated intensively again with the likelihood of more remissions. With modern aggressive therapy the possibility of a cure for leukaemia is near; at present it achieves a mean length of survival of 5 years, and there are many individuals alive over 10 years from onset. With the increased survival has come an increased prevalence of meningeal leukaemia; the bone marrow appears free from disease but the child is ill with a meningitis caused by malignant cells in the CSF. This can be effectively treated with intrathecal drugs and may be prevented by pro-phylactic irradiation early in the course of the disease.

Other reticuloendothelial system tumours

These may be associated with leukaemia, particularly in the terminal stages, but do occur independently. The commonest is lymphosarcoma. Hodgkin's disease and reticulum cell sarcoma are more rare. The mediastinum, naso-pharynx and small intestine are the usual sites in British children; in Africa the jaw is the commonest site (Burkitt's tumour).

NERVOUS SYSTEM TUMOURS

These are the second most common group of tumours.

Gliomas

Gliomas are the most important, and are usually either astrocytomas or medulloblastomas. Compared with the adult picture a much higher proportion are subtentorial. Therefore they tend to present either because of cerebellar involvement (ataxia, incoordination and nystagmus), or with raised intracranial pressure. In the young child the raised intracranial pressure will cause head enlargement and a bulging fontanelle, whilst in the older child with fused cranial sutures pain and vomiting will be earlier symptoms. Papilloedema is an important early sign.

Neuroblastomas

These arise from the sympathetic nervous system, particularly from the adrenal glands. They may present as an abdominal mass or as a result of bone or liver dissemination. An increased output of catecholamine degradation products (e.g. vanillyl-mandelic acid, VMA, HMMA) is usually present in the urine. IVP shows displacement of the kidney.

Retinoblastomas

These are uncommon intraocular neural tumours. They usually present very early in life either because of a dilated yellowish pupil or a secondary squint. They may be inherited by autosomal dominant transmission.

CONNECTIVE TISSUE TUMOURS

These include sarcomas of striped muscle, cartilage, bone and the meninges. Their presentation and course depends upon their site and degree of malignancy.

WILMS' TUMOUR (NEPHROBLASTOMA)

Nephroblastomas are embryonic renal tumours which usually present as a unilateral abdominal mass early in childhood. Microscopic haematuria occurs in up to a third of cases, but macroscopic haematuria is rare. IVP shows a distorted kidney. A combination of surgery, chemotherapy and irradiation often achieves complete cure.

RETICULOENDOTHELIOSES (HISTIOCYTOSIS X)

This is a group of rare disorders of unknown origin which are almost confined to childhood.

Eosinophilic granuloma

A localized granuloma of bone is the most benign form of histiocytosis. However, the granulomata may be generalized or progressive.

Hand–Schüller–Christian disease

This is a very rare form of the generalized disease in which skull deposits cause secondary exophthalmos, infantilism and diabetes insipidus.

Letterer–Siwe disease

The most malignant form of histiocytosis is Letterer–Siwe disease. It occurs in infants and is associated with visceral, pulmonary, skin and bone involvement.

TREATMENT OF CHILDHOOD MALIGNANCY

Specific treatment of childhood·tumours is similar to that of adults. Surgery, irradiation and chemotherapy are used singly or in combination according to the site and nature of the tumour. Every effort is made to keep the child out of hospital and leading a normal life at home and school. Many children with advanced disease can be treated on an outpatient basis provided there is good organization and flexible, sympathetic staff. Although childhood tumours are diagnosed and treated earlier than most adult tumours, their high degree of malignancy results in fewer cures.

Further reading

Nelson W.E., Vaughan V.C. & McKay R.J. (1975) Neoplasms and neoplastic-like lesions. Chapter 25, *Textbook of Paediatrics*, Saunders.

Hutchison J.H. (1975) Malignant disease in childhood. Chapter 11, *Practical Paediatric Problems*. Lloyd-Luke.

Chapter 19

ENDOCRINE AND METABOLIC DISORDERS

The essential difference between endocrine function in children and in adults is its importance in relation to physical and mental development. The relationships between the various glands, the controlling role of the pituitary, and the feed-back mechanisms, are established in prenatal life. This chapter is not intended as a comprehensive catalogue of all the endocrine diseases that can occur in children, but as an indication of those which are most important in childhood or which differ significantly in their presentation or management in children.

Hypothyroidism

Normal thyroid function is necessary for normal physical and mental growth. Congenital absence of functional thyroid tissue causes cretinism which in turn leads to dwarfing and mental deficiency unless promptly recognized and treated. Lesser degrees of hypothyroidism may develop at any time during childhood, and may present as short stature.

A cretin is not recognizable as such at birth, but suspicions may first be aroused by prolonged physiological jaundice, coming on at the usual time (2nd or 3rd day) but lasting for 2, 3 or even 4 weeks. In the absence of this clue all may appear well for a few weeks, after which lethargy, difficulty with feeding, constipation, enlargement of the tongue, and umbilical hernia become noticeable. The cry may be deep and throaty. Early diagnosis is so important that there should never be the slightest hesitation in investigating a baby on suspicion. The facial appearance is characteristic to the trained eye (Fig. 49). The most helpful tests are estimation of plasma thyroxine (T4), and X-ray of relevant epiphyses which will show marked delay. In young babies the

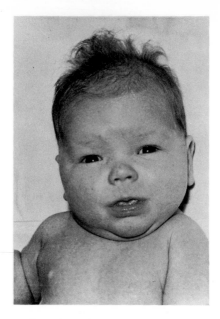

Fig. 49a. A cretin aged 4 weeks. Compare with Fig. 50b.

knee is more informative than the wrist (Appendix 5). Tests using radio-active materials are not usually necessary, but the diagnosis must be established beyond doubt as it needs life-long treatment. Treatment is with thyroxine starting with a small dose (e.g. 0.05 mg daily) and subsequently adjusting this according to the clinical response and periodic assessment of epiphyseal development. Excessive dosage will cause symptoms of thyrotoxicosis and accelerated epiphyseal development. If treatment is started within 2 or 3 months of birth and regularly maintained, there is a good chance of achieving normal physical and mental growth. The longer the delay, the poorer the prospects for mental development.

Goitre

Goitre is not common in childhood except in areas where it is

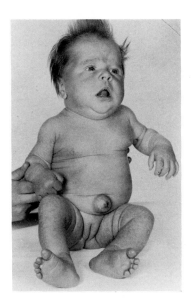

Fig. 49b. A cretin aged 4 months. She has coarse features, dry mottled skin, scanty hair and an umbilical hernia.

endemic. A baby may be born with a goitre if the mother has taken anti-thyroid drugs (including iodides) during pregnancy. Goitre with thyrotoxicosis occurs rarely in childhood. In goitrous cretinism there is a metabolic block in the synthesis of thyroid hormone due to an autosomal recessive gene. The goitre takes a few years to develop. Some enlargement of the thyroid gland in adolescent girls is very common: sometimes it becomes large enough to be called a goitre. Thyroid function is usually normal, but there may be temporary deficiency.

Diabetes mellitus

Diabetes in children is always of the ketotic, insulin-dependent variety, and diabetic children are almost always thin when first diagnosed. They usually present with a short history of polyuria, thirst and weight loss, or in pre-coma. There may be a family history of diabetes. The diagnosis is confirmed by demonstrating glucose and ketones in the urine and a high blood glucose level. The management of diabetes and diabetic coma in children is based on the same principles that apply to adult insulin-dependent diabetes. The following points are particularly relevant to children.

1 Carbohydrate intake must be carefully regulated, but the total calorie intake must be sufficient to maintain normal growth and to allow normal physical activities.

2 The child must learn to manage his own disease as soon as possible. Urine testing is now very simple, and an intelligent 7-year-old can inject his own insulin under supervision. All diabetic children should experience hypoglycaemia so that they can recognize it and know what to do about it.

3 The family must be helped to take diabetes in their stride so that it does not interfere with a normal way of life. Membership of the British Diabetic Association is helpful.

4 Diabetes in children is less stable than in adults. Periods of glycosuria are almost inevitable if hypoglycaemia is to be avoided. Insulin dosage often has to be reduced after the disease has first been brought under control. Some children have phases of requiring no insulin, but the need always returns.

The Adrenal Glands

Disorders of the adrenal gland are uncommon in children. The least rare is the adrenogenital syndrome. Total adrenocortical insufficiency (Addison's disease) is very rare. Adrenal cortical tumours may secrete androgens or oestrogens, with consequent appearance of the corresponding secondary sexual characteristics. Excess secretion of glucocorticoids and mineralocorticoids produces the clinical picture of Cushing's syndrome and may result from adenoma, carcinoma or hyperplasia of the adrenals.

The Adrenogenital syndrome

This results from a metabolic block in the synthesis of hydrocortisone, the enzyme defect occurring in individuals homozygous for an autosomal recessive gene. The fetal adrenal normally secretes hydrocortisone, and the pituitary-adrenal axis is functional in prenatal life. This disorder therefore has its origins before birth. Hydrocortisone deficiency causes increased production of ACTH by the pituitary. This causes adrenal hyperplasia and excessive production of androgens. The affected female is therefore born with an enlarged clitoris, and often labial fusion. The genitalia of affected boys look normal at birth. Many affected children lack mineralocorticoids and early in life (often about the second week) develop symptoms of salt loss—vomiting, dehydration, and collapse. This is lethal if not recognized and treated. In boys who are not salt-losers, diagnosis is likely to be delayed until it is recognized that both physical and sexual development are advancing with excessive speed (infant Hercules). Excessive androgens cause precocious pseudo-puberty, advanced bone growth and advanced epiphyseal development. In untreated cases epiphyseal fusion occurs very early and ultimate stature is therefore small.

In cases presenting as intersex, buccal smear and chromosome studies will show a normal female pattern. The diagnosis is confirmed by finding raised levels of androgen metabolites and hydrocortisone precursors (17-oxosteroids and pregnanetriol) in a 24-hour urine sample. Lowered serum sodium and chloride, with raised potassium levels, may be demonstrated in salt-losers.

Treatment is essentially the oral replacement of missing hormones. Cortisone or prednisolone are required by all patients, with additional fluorohydrocortisone for salt-losers. Precise dosage and spacing of doses is important. Inadequate control will permit excessive growth and subsequent stunting: excess steroids will stunt growth. Treatment must be lifelong, with increased dosage at times of stress. Plastic surgery may be required later to correct labial fusion or to recess a large clitoris.

Cushing's syndrome

This is most commonly seen in children who have been treated with steroids for long periods (Fig. 50). The face is fat and plethoric and there is excess facial hair. The whole body is obese and there are striae, especially on the abdomen. There may be hypertension or glycosuria. The effect of endogenous steroids on growth is variable, but a severe hazard of long-term steroid

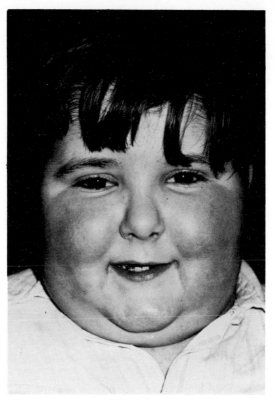

Fig. 50. Cushing's syndrome from prolonged corticosteroid therapy. The face is round, hirsute and plethoric.

administration is growth retardation. This is virtually constant if steroids are given daily and is proportionate to dose. It may be avoided by using ACTH instead; unfortunately ACTH has to be given by injection. In addition to hypertension and diabetes, which are fortunately rare, periodic checks for vertebral osteoporosis and cataract are advisable. Obesity can be minimized by calorie control.

Pituitary Disorders

Pituitary dwarfism is described on page 46.

Diabetes insipidus

This is a rare disease, resulting from either failure of the hypothalamus to produce sufficient antidiuretic hormone (ADH) or failure of the renal tubule to respond to it (nephrogenic diabetes insipidus). In either case there is marked thirst and the passage of large volumes of almost colourless urine of low specific gravity and osmolality. There is a constant danger of serious water depletion, especially in hot weather, and growth is retarded. ADH deficiency may result from a variety of intra-cranial disorders, including tumours, cysts, vascular accidents, meningitis, and Hand–Schüller–Christian disease (page 209). It may also result from an isolated hormone deficiency, genetically determined. In ADH-deficient cases, pitressin can be given by injection, as a snuff, or as a nasal spray in the form of lysine-8-vasopressin. Nephrogenic diabetes insipidus is caused by a sex-linked gene and, therefore, occurs only in males.

The Gonads

Gonadal dysgenesis and testicular feminization are dealt with elsewhere (page 55). Gonadal tumours are fortunately very rare. They may secrete androgens or oestrogens, leading to masculinization or feminization. Testicular tumours may be very small and difficult to detect.

INBORN ERRORS OF METABOLISM

This term was originally coined by Garrod to embrace three disorders, but the list has now grown to many hundreds. Most are genetically determined, usually by autosomal recessive genes, and most are extremely rare. In some, the metabolic block leads to deficiency of metabolites beyond the block and accumulation of precursors and their metabolites. Many conditions of this type lead to mental deficiency unless effective treatment can be instituted early. In others the outstanding feature is failure of reabsorption by the renal tubules of one or more substances, usually with profound metabolic consequences. Reference will only be made to a small number of conditions which illustrate general principles.

Phenylketonuria

In this disorder, which affects about 1 in 10–20,000 children born, deficiency of phenylalanine hydroxylase interferes with the conversion of phenylalanine to tyrosine. Phenylalanine levels in the blood and tissues rise, and abnormal metabolites (phenylketones) are excreted in the urine. The most serious consequence is mental defect, but there is also physical stunting, and in some cases eczema or convulsions in early infancy. The symptoms appear to be caused, at least predominantly, by the accumulation of phenylalanine and its derivatives rather than to deficiency of tyrosine. Hence, treatment by the controlled restriction of phenylalanine in the diet is helpful, and if started before symptoms develop may be dramatically beneficial. It is for this reason that programmes of population screening for the disease have been instituted in many countries. The most widely used screening procedure at present is the Guthrie test, which uses a phenylalanine-dependent strain of Bacillus subtilis as a biological indicator of serum phenylalanine concentration. It must be emphasized that this is a screening test designed to detect phenylalanine levels above 250 μmol/l: the diagnosis of phenylketonuria requires further biochemical testing of blood and urine.

Dietetic management is difficult. It requires careful biochemical control so that the serum phenylalanine is maintained within acceptable limits, and also extra vitamins. Some of the amino-acid foods are not very palatable, and as the children get older it may be difficult to control what they eat. There is good evidence that the diet need not be continued indefinitely. Some children have resumed a normal diet by 8 years of age without apparent harm. Adult phenylketonuric women have given birth to mentally retarded (though not phenylketonuric) children, presumably because of damage to the fetal brain by high levels of phenylalanine crossing the placenta. Dietetic restrictions should therefore be resumed during pregnancy.

The disorder is caused by an autosomal recessive gene. There is therefore a 25% risk of recurrence in siblings. Carriers can be detected with a reasonable degree of accuracy by a phenylalanine loading test.

Galactosaemia

Although some centres screen all infants for galactosaemia, it is not widely practised because affected babies become ill almost as soon as they begin to drink milk. A deficiency of galactose-1-phosphate-uridyl-transferase leads to accumulation of galactose in the blood and tissues and its excretion in the urine. Early symptoms are vomiting, weight loss, jaundice and hepatomegaly. Galactose (a reducing sugar) appears in the urine, provided sufficient milk feeds have been taken and retained. Hypoglycaemia may also be evident, and untreated survivors later show mental defect, cataract and cirrhosis of the liver, with hepatoma developing in some. Treatment is by the exclusion of galactose from the diet.

Babies with funny smells

Occasionally a newborn baby is noted, usually by the nursing staff, to smell strange. Some of these babies prove to have inborn errors of metabolism, the smell being due to abnormal substances in the urine. Phenylketonurics are said to have a characteristic smell, and several disorders in this group are named after the smell, e.g., maple syrup urine disease, oast-house disease, and even the odour-of-sweaty-feet syndrome. The observation of a strange smell from a baby should never be ignored.

RENAL TUBULAR DEFECTS

In this group of disorders, also genetically determined, there is failure of tubular reabsorption of one or more essential substances. Reference is made on p. 217 to nephrogenic diabetes insipidus, which is a defect of tubular reabsorption of water. Phosphate, bicarbonate, glucose and amino-acids are lost in other disorders.

Vitamin D-resistant rickets

This results from tubular loss of phosphate. The rickets develops later in childhood than nutritional rickets and may present with knock knees or bowing of the legs.

It will respond to large doses of vitamin D (25–100,000 units daily), but excessive dosage will lead to nephrocalcinosis and arterial calcification. Management is therefore difficult.

In *cystinuria* there is tubular loss of cystine (and other amino-acids), sometimes with the formation of cystine stones. This should not be confused with the more serious condition of *cystinosis*, in which cystine is stored in the tissues, there is vomiting, failure to thrive, and rickets, and the prognosis is poor; cystine crystals may be demonstrated in bone marrow and by slit-lamp examination in the cornea.

HYPOGLYCAEMIA

Hypoglycaemia is not a disease but a symptom. The maintenance of normal blood glucose levels depends upon the ingestion, absorption and metabolism of carbohydrates, and normal levels of insulin, glucocorticoids and other hormones. A wide variety of diseases may therefore be associated with hypoglycaemia. Early symptoms include hunger, irritability, pallor, sweating and tachycardia. Later symptoms include convulsions and coma. Some symptoms are probably directly due to low tissue glucose levels, others to the secretion of adrenalin which normally ensues.

Hypoglycaemia in the newborn is most often seen in low birthweight babies (especially the light-for-dates) and in the infants of diabetic mothers (page 24). Symptomatic hypoglycaemia is only exceptionally seen in starvation or malabsorption states, although blood glucose levels may be moderately low, and glucose tolerance curves flat. Amongst metabolic disorders, hypoglycaemia is a feature of galactosaemia and some types of glycogen storage disease. It may also occur during the prediabetic phase of diabetes mellitus in children. Insulin overdosage is, of course, the commonest cause of hypoglycaemia. Insulinoma is very rare.

A few infants develop hypoglycaemia after ingestion of leucine, iso-leucine or valine. The attacks therefore tend to be postprandial. Children with hypopituitarism from any cause may have hypoglycaemic episodes and are unduly sensitive to insulin.

There remains a group of children who are subject to early morning hypoglycaemic convulsions without any demonstrable underlying disease. Attacks may also occur during the daytime, possibly as a result of oversecretion of insulin.

Repeated hypoglycaemic fits may lead to brain damage and must therefore be treated vigorously. Emergency treatment consists of the intravenous injection of 50% glucose solution, which will rapidly stop fits and restore consciousness. The underlying cause must be sought and, if possible, treated. If the fundamental cause cannot be treated, diazoxide, steroids or ACTH may be helpful.

Children who are prone to spontaneous attacks in the early morning may be helped by additional protein (not carbohydrate) at bedtime.

Further reading

Hubble D. (1969) *Paediatric Endocrinology*. Blackwell Scientific Publications. Oxford.
Wilkins L. (1966) *Endocrine Disorders in Childhood*. Thomas, Illinois.

Chapter 20

THERAPEUTICS

Therapeutics is not to be regarded as synonymous with the prescription of drugs. Drugs often have an important role, but therapy includes all measures taken to relieve symptoms and to hasten recovery. In the management of medical (as distinct from surgical) conditions in children, the doctor's function is almost entirely advisory, the therapy being carried out largely by the mother at home or by nurses in hospital. Some problems need the help of specialized therapists (e.g. physiotherapists, speech therapists, occupational therapists).

GENERAL MEASURES

In any acute illness advice needs to be given about some basic aspects of management, and a worried mother caring for a sick child at home will appreciate clear guidance.

1. *Rest.* A child who feels ill will want to rest: one who feels well will not. There are very few indications for trying to enforce rest. Active disease of the heart or lungs may restrict activity, as will painful joints, but enforced inactivity will almost always do more harm than good. At home, the sofa or a comfortable chair downstairs with the TV set is more conducive to rest than bored isolation in the bedroom.

Hypoxic babies with heart or lung disease are often restless and may require sedation as well as oxygen.

2. *Temperature and humidity.* There is still a widespread fear that febrile children may suffer from chilling, and consequently parents switch on bedroom heaters and pile on blankets. Such measures can only help raise body temperature and increase discomfort and the risk of febrile convulsion in young children.

Room temperature should be comfortable (about 65°F, 18°C), preferably with an open window. High fever in a young child is an indication for active cooling by giving antipyretics, removing blankets, using fans and, if necessary, tepid sponging.

Dry air is irritating to an inflamed respiratory tract and may aggravate cough. Central heating often dries the air and this can be overcome by placing a reservoir of water by the radiator. Active humidification may give relief in laryngitis and is achieved more safely by cold humidity than by steam. High humidity can only be achieved in a tent. There is no evidence that humidification is helpful in chest infections. Even in cystic fibrosis, controlled trials have so far shown no advantage, even using ultrasonic nebulizers which produce very small droplets.

A sheltered corner of a sunny garden is a far better place than a bedroom for convalescence.

3. *Diet*. During acute illnesses, especially febrile illnesses, drinking is much more important than eating. The child should be encouraged to drink frequent small quantities of water, fruit juice or glucose drinks. A vomiting child should have a small drink after each vomit: some will return with the next vomit, but some will stay down. Fluid intake may need to be more accurately controlled and recorded in renal disease, and output should be recorded in renal disease and heart failure.

It does not matter if a sick child eats little or nothing for a few days. Parents should be told that the lost weight will soon be regained. Appetite is a good guide, and a little of what the child fancies will probably do good. Returning appetite is a good sign of returning health. In some renal disorders, diabetes mellitus, coeliac disease and inborn errors of metabolism, more strictly controlled diets are needed.

4. *Isolation*. Children with infectious diseases nursed at home do not necessarily need to be isolated. Measles and chicken pox are highly infectious before the spots appear, and siblings are probably already infected when the rash develops. With rubella, the risk to pregnant women must be remembered. Infective hepatitis is unpleasant, especially in adults. Barrier nursing with disinfection of excreta is advisable at home as in hospital.

5. *Schoolwork*. To miss any substantial time from school may set back a child's educational progress, especially if this happens around the time of crucial examinations. In most hospitals

teachers are made available by Education Authorities to work on children's wards. At home, teachers are usually glad to provide schoolwork and will sometimes call in to help with problems. For children confined to their homes for long periods, regular home teaching may be provided. Children who have been ill should be allowed back to school as soon as possible, if necessary on a part-time basis initially, but physical activities (games and PE) may need to be postponed for longer.

DRUGS

When these general points have been attended to, more often than not it will be appropriate to prescribe one or more drugs. In spite of the enormous number of drugs and compounds available, the wise doctor will confine his prescribing to a relatively small number of drugs with which he is familiar. The newest drug is not necessarily the best, and is certainly the one of which there is least experience. An old remedy is not necessarily a bad one. Experienced doctors find that they can treat all but the most obscure conditions with fewer than fifty drugs.

The prescription of a drug for a patient is often done with little thought at all, but if medicine is to be practised at its best, it demands a 10-point catechism.

1. *Is a drug necessary?* Am I treating a symptom or the underlying disease, or am I prescribing a placebo to make anxious parents or myself feel better? Is this a virus infection, because if so I might be wiser to avoid antibiotics?

2. *If so, which one?* If an antibiotic, what organisms are likely to be involved and what will be effective against them? What drug has the best chance of doing good without doing harm? Prefer a familiar drug to an unfamiliar. Other things being equal, economize. The use of official names may save money.

3. *Which preparation shall I use?* Try to find something palatable for young children. Don't order capsules for babies unless it is permissible to put the contents in a spoon. Some young children prefer tablets: some old ones prefer medicines. Ask the mother.

4. *What route of administration?* Don't give injections if they can be avoided, *but* they may be necessary if the child is vomiting or if

it is necessary to achieve high tissue levels quickly. If there is peripheral circulatory failure, drugs given by intramuscular injection may be absorbed slowly. If there is serious infection (meningitis, septicaemia) give antibiotics intravenously to begin with.

5. *How much, how often, for how long?* There is no infallible formula for calculating dosage for children. The younger the child, the more critical the dose (especially the newborn baby). There is a big margin of safety for some drugs, but very little for others, such as digoxin. Therefore, put the child's age or date of birth on the prescription. This gives the pharmacist a chance to check the dose. Frequency of administration depends on the duration of action of the drug. Do not disturb sleep unnecessarily. Arrange an infant's drug schedule to fit in with the feeding schedule (i.e. avoid ordering 6-hourly drugs and 4-hourly feeds). Remember to specify the duration of treatment.

6. *Is the drug compatible with the patient?* Is there any history of drug allergy or other untoward reaction? Has he any disorder which limits the use of any drugs (e.g. glucose-6-phosphate dehydrogenase deficiency).

7. *Is the drug compatible with other drugs?* If two or more drugs are being given, ensure that they do not inhibit or potentiate one another. Be especially careful of mixing drugs for intravenous administration.

8. *Have I written the prescription legibly?*

9. *Have I given any necessary instructions about the administration of the drug or its storage?*

10. *Have I given any necessary warning* of side effects, whether harmless (e.g. dark stools with iron) or serious?

A general indication of the drugs appropriate for the treatment of common conditions will be found in the other chapters of this book, but some comments on common prescribing problems are included here. In most clinical situations there is no one line of treatment that is undoubtedly superior to all others and you may therefore meet a bewildering variety of therapeutic approaches amongst your medical teachers. Sometimes you may meet direct conflict, one teacher advising you never to do something that another habitually does. Have courage and ask the reason why.

Prescribing for the newborn

Very few drugs are needed for the treatment of neonatal disease, and others are positively harmful. Many of the metabolic functions of the liver and the excretory capacity of the kidneys take a week or so to develop fully. During this time very high blood levels of drugs may be achieved on relatively low dosage. This is especially true of the pre-term infant. Chloramphenicol, sulphonamides, tetracyclines, lincomycin and novobiocin should be avoided altogether. Serious infections at this age are usually caused by Gram-negative bacteria (chiefly *E. coli*) and are best treated with gentamicin combined with ampicillin *or* penicillin. Nalorphine (1 mg IV or IM) is an antidote to morphine and pethidine. Stimulants such as ethamivan are sometimes used in infants with respiratory depression. Irritability and convulsions due to cerebral problems may be controlled with phenobarbitone or chloral hydrate, but if due to metabolic disturbances (e.g. hypoglycaemia) appropriate correction must be made.

Oxygen is a powerful therapeutic weapon for good or ill. In the severely asphyxiated newborn, endotracheal oxygen is the most pressing need. In respiratory and some cardiac problems the intelligent use of oxygen is crucial. Excessive concentrations of oxygen can damage the eyes, the brain and the lungs. Monitoring is therefore essential, at least of the inspired air and preferably of arterial oxygen saturation.

Digoxin must always be used with care, especially in the newborn and most of all in the pre-term infant. The margin between therapeutic and toxic doses is narrow and in the event of overdosage there is no effective antidote. Calculate the dose with care and watch hawk-eyed for early signs of toxicity.

Iron and vitamin supplements are needed by all pre-term babies. It is not *necessary* to start them before 6 weeks, and little iron is absorbed before this time, but it is *traditional* to start them before the baby is discharged home.

Antibiotics

If there are infections in paradise the causative organism will be known every time and there will be available an antibiotic which kills that organism and no others. In this life we must make an intelligent guess at the organism (the laboratory may give us help after a day or two) and decide what chemotherapy is appropriate. If the infection is certainly or probably viral (measles, influenza, laryngitis) antibiotics are not needed. The notion of 'preventing secondary bacterial infection' is not valid in children. In some bacterial infections, especially bacillary dysentery, there is good evidence that antibiotics do harm. There may be genuine diagnostic uncertainties, as between bronchiolitis (viral) and bronchopneumonia (viral or bacterial) in infants.

If swabs or samples of urine, faeces, blood or CSF are needed for culture, take them before starting antibiotics. Swabs, unless of frank pus, need to be taken thoroughly, transported expeditiously and incubated promptly.

Some antibiotics cause diarrhoea, others (especially ampicillin) cause rashes. Such symptoms often settle in spite of continuation of the drug. Babies given broad-spectrum antibiotics often develop oral thrush (moniliasis). Tetracyclines should be avoided under the age of 7 years because they damage and discolour the teeth.

There is no need to give any vitamin supplements with courses of antibiotics lasting less than a month. In paediatric practice, therefore, vitamin B supplements are only needed with chemotherapy in tuberculosis.

If an unnecessary antibiotic has been started, stop it as soon as possible.

Anticonvulsants

The drugs appropriate to the treatment of different forms of epilepsy are discussed in Chapter 6.

Phenobarbitone is often tolerated well by children but may make them hyperactive. Blood levels fall after the first week or two of treatment because the induction of liver enzymes leads to more rapid inactivation. If half the calculated dose is given for the first fortnight, early side effects will be minimized. If facilities are available for determining serum levels, these provide a helpful indication of the adequacy of the dose and reliability of administration.

Phenytoin nearly always causes some gum hypertrophy, but this subsides when the drug is stopped. Hirsutism may also occur. Megaloblastic anaemia responsive to folates is a rare complication, although depression of folate levels is common.

Changes in drugs or in dosage for epileptic children should be made gradually. Push each drug to the limit of tolerance before abandoning it. Try to avoid giving several drugs simultaneously.

Sedatives and tranquillizers

It should only be exceptionally necessary to prescribe these drugs for children. The use of hypnotics for sleep disturbances is described on page 105. Tranquillizers are sometimes needed for children with behaviour disorders, but they should only be used as an adjunct to attempts to determine and influence the cause of the misbehaviour. Tricyclic anti-depressants are sometimes useful in the management of enuresis.

Steroids

Cortisone and its many relatives may be used either locally or systemically, for short-term or long-term treatment.

Local steroids include many preparations for the treatment of skin conditions (e.g. betamethasone for eczema) and steroids for inhalation (e.g. beclamethasone for asthma). The quantities of steroid absorbed from these preparations appears to be minimal and long-term use does not cause a cushingoid state.

Short-term oral or parenteral steroids are valuable in the treatment of severe asthmatic attacks, overwhelming infections and allergic reactions. In this critical situation big doses should be given, but can soon be stopped.

Medium-term (a few weeks) oral steroids are used to induce remissions in leukaemia, the nephrotic syndrome and some autoimmune disorders. During treatment excessive weight gain, plethora and hirsutism commonly develop, but subside when treatment is stopped. More serious side effects are rare.

Long-term (months or years) oral steroids are rarely needed and always cause side effects, notably stunting of growth, except when they are being used as replacement therapy. Regular checks of weight, height, blood pressure, urine (for diabetes), eyes (for cataract) and spine X-ray (for osteoporosis) should be made. Stunting of height may be reduced by giving intermittent (e.g. alternate day) steroids, or by using ACTH or tetracosactrin which must be injected. Excessive weight gain can be prevented by calorie control.

Salicylates

In paediatrics, salicylates are used either in modest dosage for a short period or in heroic doses for a longer period. The first is an effective way to relieve pains and reduce fever. If soluble aspirin is given in a sensible dose for not more than 2 or 3 days at a time, it is a safe drug at any age.

In acute rheumatism (rheumatic fever) salicylates have a specific effect, but should be given in maximal dosage for maximal relief (see page 168). They are also the drug of first choice for rheumatoid arthritis, and here again big doses may be necessary. In children with capillary or platelet defects salicyates should be avoided. Paracetamol may be used instead.

Further reading

Burland W.L. & Laurance B.M. (eds) (1972) *The Therapeutic Choice in Paediatrics.* Churchill Livingstone, Edinburgh and London.

Chapter 21

IMMUNITY, IMMUNIZATION AND SPECIFIC FEVERS

Most illness in childhood is infective, and an important activity in the early life of every individual is meeting and establishing immunity to a wide variety of infecting organisms. Immunological mechanisms in childhood are essentially the same as in adults but are not fully developed at birth. Cellular immunity is effective from birth: for the first two or three years of life, lymphocytes predominate over polymorphs in the circulating blood, but the total white cell count is relatively high (page 199). Pus can be formed at any age. Humoral immunity is slower to develop. Maternal IgG is transferred across the placenta from early fetal life and in the full-term infant approximates to adult levels. This conveys passive immunity to a number of common infections, including measles, rubella and mumps. In contrast, the larger molecules of IgM do not cross the placenta and the neonate is therefore fully susceptible to bacterial infections including pertussis. The fetus is capable of making its own IgM in response to intrauterine infection, e.g. rubella, but synthesis of other immunoglobulins gets off to a rather sluggish start after birth. A reasonable level of humoral immunity is established by the age of 6–9 months (Fig. 51).

Pre-term babies have relatively low levels of circulating immunoglobulins, and are particularly susceptible to infection. Total immunoglobulin levels in all infants reach their lowest at about 3–4 months of age which is another susceptible period. In older children, recurrent infections are rarely due to immunological deficiencies. Poor social conditions and debilitating diseases such as cystic fibrosis or congenital heart disease may predispose to infection. Recurrent skin infections may be associated with nasal carriage of Staph. pyogenes, and recurrent urinary infections with congenital anomalies of the renal tract or vesicouretic reflux. Rarely, however, repeated infections, especially of the skin and lungs, may be due to some defect of the defence mechanisms. Cellular immunity may be impaired by deficiency of granulocytes (seen especially in children undergoing treatment with cytotoxic drugs) or by qualitative defects of the white cells, as in chronic granulomatous disease. Hypo-gamma-globulinaemia is encountered in a number of rare disorders.

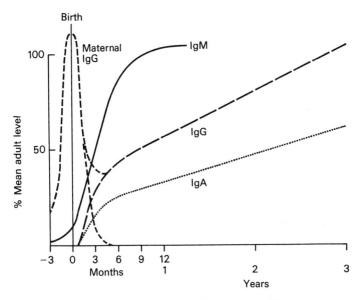

Fig. 51.   Immunoglobulin levels in early life.

IMMUNIZATION

As infectious diseases account for a large part of the mortality and morbidity of early childhood it is logical to institute whatever preventive measures are available. Table 14 shows the programme of immunization currently recommended for children in the U.K. In determining such a schedule, two basic decisions need to be made. (1) Against what diseases should a child be protected?

Table 14. Schedule of immunization procedures

Age	Prophylactic	Notes
During the first year of life	Diph/Tet/Pert. and oral polio vaccine. (First dose.)	The earliest age at which the first dose should be given is 3 months, but a better general immunological response can be expected if the first dose is delayed to 6 months of age.
	Diph/Tet/Pert. and oral polio vaccine. (Second dose.) Preferably after an interval of 6 to 8 weeks.	
	Diph/Tet/Pert. and oral polio vaccine. (Third dose.) Preferably after an interval of 6 months.	
During the second year of life	Measles vaccination. Not less than 3 weeks after last immunization.	Live measles vaccine should not be given to children below the age of nine months since it usually fails to immunize such children owing to the presence of maternally transmitted antibodies.
At 5 years of age or school entry	Diph/Tet and oral polio vaccine or Diph/Tet/Polio vaccine	These may be given, if desired, at 3 years of age to children entering nursery schools, attending day nurseries or living in children's homes.
Between 10 and 13 years of age	BCG vaccine	For tuberculin-negative children
Between 11 and 14 years of age	Rubella vaccine	For girls
At 15 to 19 years of age or on leaving school	Polio vaccine (oral or inactivated) Tetanus toxoid	

This requires a balance of the probabilities of him (a) catching it, (b) suffering death or disability from it, and (c) the dangers and effectiveness of the immunizing procedure. The more common and the more dangerous the disease, and the safer the immunization, the greater the need. (2) At what age should immunization be done? This depends upon the age of susceptibility of the child and the age at which he can best respond to the vaccine. There is often a conflict here, as in the case of pertussis. The greatest danger of the disease is in the first six months of life, but the immunological response is poor before 6 months of age.

Diphtheria

This has become an excessively rare disease in Britain, whereas at the turn of the century it was a major cause of death in childhood. The continuance of this happy state depends upon continuing immunization of as many infants as possible. The toxoid scarcely ever causes any disturbance and there are no contra-indications.

Tetanus

Tetanus is rare, but the mortality rate is still substantial and routine immunization is wise. Tetanus toxoid is safe and effective. This contrasts with anti-tetanus serum (ATS) which is prepared from horse serum and frequently causes reactions, some of which are serious and a few fatal. The value of ATS is limited because antibodies to it are rapidly developed and it is likely that any dose except the first received by an individual is rapidly inactivated. ATS should be reserved for the treatment of tetanus.

Pertussis

Pertussis vaccine, the third component of triple vaccine, is the only one of the three to cause any disturbance of health. Minor reactions are common, restlessness, fever or transient screaming episodes coming on a few hours after the injection. They last a few hours. Occasionally the temperature rises high enough to cause a febrile convulsion. It has been suggested that pertussis vaccine may cause neurological damage (infantile spasms and mental defect) but the relationship is still unproven. Nevertheless it is recommended that it should not be given to infants with any evidence of disordered brain function (e.g. fits or cerebral palsy), or to a child who has had a previous reaction to pertussis immunization.

Poliomyelitis

Poliomyelitis vaccine is usually given in the oral form (Sabin vaccine) which contains live virus. Side-effects are practically unknown and there are no contra-indications in childhood. It is highly effective.

Smallpox

Vaccination for smallpox was included in the recommended schedule for infants until 1971, when the declining incidence of smallpox in endemic areas of the world reduced the danger of smallpox in Britain below the danger of vaccination. It is no longer routinely recommended in Britain. Minor complications include secondary infection, secondary vaccination by transfer of virus to a second site, and generalized vaccinia. The most serious complications are encephalitis, which complicates about 1 in every 100,000 vaccinations, and eczema vaccinatum. The latter is likely to occur if infants with eczema are exposed to vaccinia virus, either by direct vaccination (which should never be done in eczematous children) or by accidental transfer of virus from another vaccinated individual.

Measles

Measles vaccination with a live attenuated vaccine has been introduced relatively recently. It appears to be safe and effective. A mild measles-like illness may occur after the immunization. Antibodies persist for at least 10 years and it is likely that the protection is life long.

Rubella

This is not a danger except to the embryo. In Britain vaccination is recommended for girls aged 11–14 years, and to selected adult females who are shown to be non-immune. The duration of immunity is not yet known but is not less than 7 years.

BCG

BCG vaccination gives substantial protection against tuberculosis. It is injected intradermally over the region of insertion of the deltoid muscle, and is followed 3–6 weeks later by local erythema, induration and sometimes ulceration. The axillary glands may enlarge and be painful. The local signs go in 2–6 months. The use of BCG varies greatly in different countries. In Britain school children have a tuberculin test at the age of 10–12 years and the 90% who are tuberculin negative are subsequently given BCG. Babies are given BCG during the neonatal period if anyone in the immediate family has had T.B. In some countries BCG is given routinely to all infants.

SPECIFIC FEVERS

The main clinical features of the common infectious diseases of childhood together with their incubation periods and important complications are listed in Table 15. The following paragraphs describe the aspects of these diseases which are important in childhood.

Measles

This usually presents with respiratory catarrh, misery, fever and a rash. Less frequent presentations include febrile convulsion and epistaxis. Sometimes the prodrome appears prolonged, with unexplained, intermittent fever. A prodromal rash, quite unlike a measles rash, may appear at about the time of appearance of Koplik's spots. Otitis media and bronchopneumonia are common complications: encephalitis affects about 1 in 1000 cases. In the absence of complications, antibiotics are not indicated.

Rubella

Rubella may also present with epistaxis. In general the illness is very mild and there are vitually no complications; the arthralgia of the hands so common in adolescent and adult females does not affect children.

Table 15. Common infectious diseases

Disease	Incubation period (days)*	Main features	Important complications	Laboratory findings
Measles	7–*10*–12	Misery, fever, catarrh, cough, conjunctivitis; Koplik's spots; blotchy, red rash on face and trunk	Pneumonia Otitis media Encephalitis	Rise in antibody titre
Rubella	10–*18*–21	Upper respiratory catarrh; macular or erythematous rash, chiefly on trunk; cervical adenopathy	Virtually none in childhood Encephalitis very rare	Virus culture from stool or nose Rise in antibody titre
Chickenpox	10–*14*–21	Rash on trunk, perineum and scalp; papules, vesicles, pustules, scabs; fever at pustular stage	Conjunctival lesions Encephalitis	
Mumps	14–*18*–28	Parotitis, sometimes involvement of other salivary glands	Meningitis Pancreatitis Orchitis after puberty	Virus from saliva Rise in antibody titre Lymphocytosis
Whooping-cough	7–*10*–14	Upper respiratory catarrh; paroxysmal cough with vomiting. Modified greatly by immunization	Pneumonia Lobar collapse Convulsions Haemorrhage (nose, eyes, brain)	B. pertussis from cough plate or per-nasal swab Lymphocytosis + +
Scarlet fever	1–*3*–7	Tonsillitis (pharyngitis); diffuse, erythematous rash chiefly on trunk; sore, coated tongue; circumoral pallor	Otitis media Rheumatic fever Acute nephritis	Gp. A haem. strep. from throat Rise in ASO titre

* outer figures = range, centre figure = usual

Chicken pox (varicella)

This is usually a mild disease. The differential daignosis is from papular urticaria (page 180) which, if scratched and infected, also presents papules, vesicles, pustules and scabs. However, the lesions in chicken pox are predominantly on the trunk, whilst papular urticaria is peripherally distributed. Mild cases of small-pox may cause diagnostic difficulty, but again the lesions are predominantly peripheral. Complications are rare. Chicken pox encephalitis presents as ataxia a week or so after the rash has appeared; the prognosis is good.

Mumps

This is most commonly confused with cervical adenitis. The exact location of the swelling, the fact that it is nearly always bilateral, the swelling of the orifice of the parotid ducts, and absence of any cause for cervical adenitis, should make the diagnosis clear. Presternal oedema has been a feature of mumps in some epidemics. Meningitis is a serious complication (page 72). Pancreatitis and orchitis are rare before puberty.

Whooping-cough (pertussis)

Whooping-cough is a serious disease in the very young infant, and unpleasant at all ages. Babies with pertussis do not whoop, but the cough is paroxysmal and associated with vomiting. The cough is worse at night in children who are upright during the day. Severe spasms may lead to capillary rupture, which only rarely occurs in the brain, or may lead to hypoxia sufficient to cause a convulsion. Lobar collapse is not uncommon and may lead to bronchiectasis if not detected and treated. Encephalopathy is rare. In children who have been immunized the disease tends to be mild, the whoop absent, and there may be no lymphocytosis: the diagnosis is then easily missed.

Scarlet fever

This has become a very rare disease since the introduction of penicillin.

Roseola infantum (exanthem subitum)

Roseola infantum is a mild disease of infants and young children, common outside hospital but rarely severe enough to need admission. Catarrhal symptoms and fever for 2 or 3 days are followed by the abrupt appearance of light red, discrete macules on the trunk. As the rash appears, the fever rapidly settles and the child is greatly improved. A few days later, the illness is over.

Glandular fever (infectious mononucleosis)

Glandular fever may be regarded as a disease or as a syndrome, since a similar clinical picture may result from infection by several viruses or by Toxoplasma gondii. The onset is gradual, with malaise, anorexia and low-grade fever for 1–2 weeks, after which more specific signs may develop.

1   Lymphadenopathy—multiple, firm, discrete, non-tender glands especially in the neck. They never suppurate.
2   Splenomegaly.
3   Pharyngitis.
4   Rash in some cases, macular or urticarial.
5   Jaundice—resulting from an associated hepatitis or from enlarged glands in the porta hepatis.
6   Meningeal involvement, with headache, stiff neck, and raised cells and protein in the CSF.

In classical glandular fever the peripheral blood shows an increased number of mononuclear cells (lymphocytes and monocytes) with atypical lymphocytes ('glandular fever cells'). The Paul–Bunnell test (sheep's red-cell agglutination) is positive. However, the same clinical picture may present with a negative Paul–Bunnell Test.

Infectious hepatitis (catarrhal jaundice)

This is the commonest cause of jaundice in children over the age of 3 years. It tends to be milder in children than in adults. There is a prodromal period lasting about a week, in which malaise, anorexia, abdominal pain and nausea predominate, before jaundice appears. The liver is tender and a little enlarged. The stools are pale, the urine dark, and urine testing reveals the presence of urobilinogen and bile pigment. Urobilinogen may be detected in the pre-icteric stage and may be the sole diagnostic clue in the mildest cases in which clinical jaundice does not develop. Serum bilirubin levels are raised, with roughly equal parts conjugated and free; transaminase levels are raised, and flocculation tests are abnormal.

Differential diagnosis in the pre-icteric and non-icteric cases is from other causes of abdominal pain and vomiting. Once jaundice has developed, diagnosis is not difficult. Complications are very rare. Jaundice usually fades in 1–2 weeks but exceptionally persists for months.

Cross-infection should be prevented as far as possible by care in handling stools and by conscientious hand-washing by the patient and attendants. However, infectivity is greatest before jaundice appears and it is quite common to have more than one case in a household. Diet may be dictated by appetite, which usually means omitting fatty foods and eggs initially. In the average case the child will be confined to bed for a week and kept off school for 2–3 weeks.

TUBERCULOSIS

Tuberculosis is a social indicator disease, being common wherever poverty, malnutrition and overcrowding are prevalent, and rare where standards of hygiene and nutrition are good. In the developing countries of the world tuberculosis appears in forms which were common in Britain 50 years ago. The chief sources of infection are adults with sputum-positive pulmonary tuberculosis, and milk from infected cattle. Prevention depends first upon general improvement in socio-economic conditions, and second upon specific measures including the prompt recognition and treatment of infectious adults, BCG immunization, tuberculin testing of cattle and pasteurization of milk. Mass miniature radiography is of most value where the disease is most prevalent.

The initial infection is in the lungs if conveyed by droplets, in the bowel if conveyed by milk. The first site of infection is known as the primary *focus*: the primary *complex* comprises the primary focus and the enlarged lymph nodes draining it. Spread of infection beyond the local nodes may result in tubercle bacilli reaching the blood stream, causing either tuberculous septicaemia (miliary TB) or infection of distant organs (meninges, kidneys, bones and joints). Tuberculous cervical lymph nodes are thought to be infected via the tonsils.

In Britain now childhood tuberculosis is uncommon. In 1972 in England and Wales there were 12 childhood deaths from TB of which 10 were from tuberculous meningitis. Primary complexes in the lung are seen more often in immigrant children from Asia than in others, and tuberculous meningitis is a rare disease.

Pulmonary Tuberculosis

The child with pulmonary TB must not be visualized as an emaciated invalid coughing up blood. Haemoptysis is excessively rare, and systemic symptoms such as fever and weight loss are exceptional. Symptoms are usually minor—malaise, anorexia, cough—and many children with TB traced through their contact with infected adults are completely symptom-free. Diagnosis is based on the X-ray appearances and a positive tuberculin test. Sputum is not usually present, but tubercle bacilli may be recovered from gastric washings. The ESR is usually slightly elevated if the disease is active.

Tuberculous meningitis

This disease which was universally fatal before the discovery of streptomycin is still a serious disease, especially in infancy. It most commonly affects young children and the onset is insidious so that there is usually a history of weight loss or poor weight gain. Initially there is vague malaise, anorexia and perhaps slight fever. After a few days evidence of meningeal involvement is shown by headache, drowsiness, irritability and neck stiffness. If the diagnosis is not made at this stage, convulsions, pareses and impairment of consciousness supervene. The clinical signs are those of meningitis (see p. 72). In addition, choroidal tubercles may be visible as small yellow lesions close to retinal arteries. A careful search must be made with the pupils dilated because the detection of choroidal tubercles is the quickest way of making a certain diagnosis. The CSF may be hazy, and a cobweb clot forms if the fluid is left undisturbed for 24 hours. The cell content is raised, though not extremely so. The cells are predominantly lymphocytes, but polymorphs may predominate in the early stages. Protein is raised: glucose is usually low, but not as low as in pyogenic meningitis. Tubercle bacilli may be seen on suitably stained films of CSF, but their absence does not exclude the diagnosis. Culture and guinea-pig inoculation take several weeks. A chest X-ray may show a localized lesion or miliary lesions. In very sick children the tuberculin test may be negative, and this should never be allowed to exclude the diagnosis. The differential diagnosis is from pyogenic and benign lymphocytic meningitis.

Cervical adenopathy

Tuberculous neck glands are now rare in Britain. Usually a single gland or group of glands is affected, on one side of the neck. The gland is firm (unless caseating), partially fixed and not especially tender. The tuberculin test is positive. The differential diagnosis is from Hodgkin's disease, and infection by anonymous myco-bacteria, a group of organisms related to the tubercle bacillus but less virulent. Enlarged glands associated with recurrent tonsillitis are usually bilateral, fairly soft, and mobile, though occasionally they form a localized abscess requiring chemotherapy or drainage.

Management

Regardless of the site the management can be divided into three parts.
1 Notification of the case to the Area Environmental Health Specialist so that contacts can be immunized and possible sources of infection identified.
2 Anti-tuberculous drugs. PAS and isoniazid form the basis of treatment in most cases. If there are systemic signs, such as fever, weight loss or a high ESR, streptomycin may be given for the first few weeks of treatment. This is always necessary in miliary TB and tuberculous meningitis, but only in a minority of children with pulmonary disease. Treatment should be continued for about 2 years.
3 General management. Children should not be admitted to

hospital or kept off school without good reason. A pulmonary primary complex is rarely infectious, and isolation is often unnecessary. If nutrition is unsatisfactory, it should be improved.

The combination of preventive and therapeutic measures is now so effective that the childhood mortality from tuberculosis has shrunk almost to vanishing point, but only continuing vigilance will keep it this way.

Further reading

Forfar J.O. & Arneil G.C. (eds) (1973) Diseases due to infection. Chapter 22, *Textbook of Paediatrics*. Churchill Livingstone, Edinburgh and London.

Chapter 22

ACCIDENTS AND POISONING

The health of British children is now so good that accidents account for the loss of more lives amongst school children than does any disease. Road traffic accidents are often fatal, as are severe burns, and accidental poisoning occasionally kills. Almost more tragic are the children left with permanent brain damage after severe head injuries, and those with extensive scarring from burns and scalds. Drowning is another important cause of child death.

Accidents are most common at age 1–4 years, when children are mobile but not yet responsible for their actions. They are more common amongst boys than girls. By the age of 11 one in four children has experienced a serious accident. The risk of accident is obviously influenced by social circumstances. Watchful parents, enclosed gardens, fireguards, stair-gates, locked medicine cupboards, and clothes of non flammable materials will prevent many accidents. The child of a large family in an industrial slum, on the street much of the day and ostensibly supervised by another child only marginally older, is at great hazard. A reduction in mortality and morbidity from accidents can only be brought about by better education of children, parents and drivers about safety; by legislation to minimize the opportunities for accidents; and by improved design of towns and homes.

HEAD INJURY

The management of head injuries in children calls for some experience. On the one hand, scalps split easily and bleed profusely, but the quantity of blood may cause unjustifiable alarm. On the other hand, some apparently trivial injuries are associated with intracranial bleeding that only becomes apparent after an interval of time. A history of unconsciousness, however brief, should be regarded seriously. Pallor, vomiting and sleepiness can occur after quite minor injuries, but should settle within an hour or two. Progressive symptoms or the appearance of abnormal neurological signs suggest intracranial injury.

It is customary to have a skull X-ray taken, but a linear fracture without displacement may be unimportant, whilst intracranial bleeding may occur without a fracture. In any case of doubt it is wiser to admit a child with a head injury to hospital for 24 hours' observation, which will include frequent recording of pulse and respiratory rates, blood pressure, level of consciousness and pupillary size and reactions. If there is any suggestion of intracranial bleeding, the opinion of a neurosurgeon should be sought without delay.

BURNS AND SCALDS

Scalds are caused by hot fluids and cause predominantly loss of the epidermis only, with blistering and peeling. Burns are caused by direct contact with very hot objects or by the clothes catching fire and result in full thickness skin loss. The death rate from burns and scalds varies directly with the proportion of the total body surface involved. Loss of skin surface leads to loss of fluid and shock. If more than 10% of the body surface is involved (Fig. 52), intravenous fluid therapy will be required. Burns involving 50% or more of the body surface carry a grave prognosis, although children have survived much more extensive burns than this. The management of scalds involves the correction of fluid loss, the prevention of infection and the relief of pain. Burns require in addition skin grafting where there has been full thickness skin loss. As a general rule, burns and scalds are more serious than they seem, and hospital admission is advisable for all but the most trivial.

POISONING

The accidental swallowing of drugs and household fluids by young children is extremely common, but remarkably few of them be-

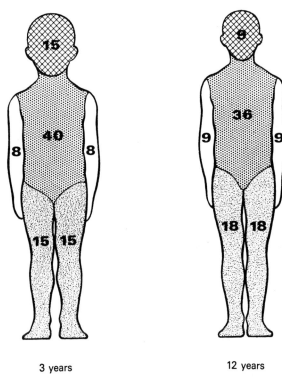

3 years   12 years

Fig. 52. Skin surface areas at 3 years and 12 years of age. The figures indicate the percentage of total body surface represented by each part.

come ill and mortality is very low. The great majority are 2- and 3-year-olds who are sufficiently agile to get hold of things to swallow, but not old enough to appreciate the potential dangers. Occasionally younger babies are fed with poisonous substances by their toddler siblings. If older children in the prepubertal-adolescent age range swallow poisonous substances (usually drugs) this is indicative of an emotional upset. Most often it is done as a gesture of defiance without serious intent to commit suicide, but some children are pathologically depressed at this age, and the advice of a child psychiatrist should always be sought when children of this age have swallowed poison.

The things that children swallow are numberless, but fall into three main categories:

1 Tablets and medicines. Aspirin is the most frequently swallowed drug because it is in every home. Sleeping tablets, tranquillizers and iron are also high on the list.

2 Household and horticultural fluids. Bleach, turpentine, paraffin (kerosene), cleaning fluids and weedkillers form the bulk of this group.

3 Berries and seeds. Laburnum tops the list, with deadly nightshade and toadstools featuring prominently.

The basis of treatment of poisoning is to minimize absorption, to promote excretion and to combat symptoms. With some important exceptions, the stomach should be emptied by the most efficient means available unless more than 6 hours have elapsed since the poison was swallowed. For children, most authorities favour induced emesis rather than gastric lavage. It is more effective in removing solid matter (e.g. whole tablets or berries), it is less unpleasant for the child, and it occupies less nursing time. Emesis usually follows the administrations of 20 mls ipecacuanha syrup in orange juice, repeated if necessary. Gastric lavage may be needed if emesis does not occur, or if the child is unconscious. The exceptions to the rule of emesis are (a) caustics, such as bleach or acids, which may be presumed from burning around the mouth if there is no adequate history, and (b) hydrocarbons such as turpentine and paraffin. In the case of caustics, the danger of gastric perforation is increased by emesis or lavage: hydrocarbons do little harm in the gastro-intestinal tract, but inhalation of vomit may seriously damage the lungs.

Absorption may be discouraged by diluting the poison (milk is good and usually available), by giving an absorbent agent such as activated charcoal, or by giving a specific antidote (e.g. desferrioxamine in iron poisoning). Excretion may be encouraged by the use of purgatives or forced diuresis in selected cases. Supportive treatment in severe cases includes mechanical ventilation for respiratory depression; correction of acid-base balance in aspirin poisoning; and exchange transfusion or peritoneal dialysis in selected cases.

It is usually advisable to admit poisoned children to hospital for observation for at least a few hours. Most major centres now concentrate the management of serious poisoning in specialized units, and a few provide advisory and information services by telephone.

Chronic lead poisoning

Lead poisoning is uncommon in Britain. Lead water pipes have been largely replaced by copper, and drinking water is drawn from main supplies rather than storage tanks. Modern paints for interior decoration contain very little lead, and the British climate does not readily bring to mind the thought of peeling paint on the railings of a sun-baked verandah. Nevertheless, some risks still exist. Amateurs may use lead paints for home decorating or painting cots: lead dust may lie in the vicinity of smelting works or come home on the clothes of lead workers: and disused car batteries are a cheap, if dangerous, form of domestic fuel. Lead may be absorbed by ingestion, inhalation, or through the skin. There may be a history of the child eating dirt or paint (pica).

Poisoning is usually chronic and the onset of symptoms is insidious. Early symptoms include abdominal colic, pallor, anaemia, irritability, anorexia and disturbed sleep. Later symptoms are predominantly neurological, including encephalopathy, neuropathy and convulsions. Permanent brain damage may result in mental deficiency. If the onset is more acute, encephalopathic features tend to predominate.

The most difficult part of diagnosis is considering the possibility of lead poisoning. Investigation will then include the measurement of lead levels in blood and urine; estimation of urinary coproporphyrins; X-rays of long bones seeking dense zones at the metaphyses; X-rays of abdomen for opacities within the bowel; and examination of blood films for evidence of hypochromic anaemia and basophil stippling of red cells. Raised lead levels indicate exposure to lead, but not necessarily poisoning. In encephalopathy, there may be raised protein and lymphocytes in the CSF.

Management depends upon the severity of symptoms and will not be described in detail. The principles are:
1 To identify and eliminate the source of poisoning.
2 To encourage the excretion of lead (except in mild cases)

by the use of EDTA (ethylene diamine tetra-acetic acid; calcium versenate), penicillamine or BAL (British anti-lewisite).

3   To treat major symptoms (convulsions, colic).

NON-ACCIDENTAL INJURY ('battered babies')

It may seem inappropriate to discuss deliberate injury to children in a chapter on accidents, but in spite of much publicity about battered babies doctors still fail to recognize the true nature of some childhood injuries. Although children of any age may be physically abused, babies under 6 months are especially vulnerable. The true incidence is unknown but is certainly not less than 5 per 1000 children.

There are probably 4000 children in Britain who are injured through purposeful acts of their parents each year, and of these about 400 die. At least an equal number suffer permanent injury leading to mental impairment or neurological abnormality (cerebral palsy).

No parents are immune to the possibility of striking their child in anger, but certain features commonly underlie child abuse.

The parents have often been subject to cruelty in their own childhood. The injured child cries excessively and is over-demanding. The home is overcrowded so that parents and children are constantly on top of one another. Father may be on shift-work and attempting to sleep when the family is awake.

Injury and neglect are closely associated and are both indications of parental inadequacy. The child with non-accidental injury may, therefore, also show evidence of poor standards of hygiene or nutrition, although most are well-fed. The family may already be known to the health visitor as in need of supervision. In other cases one child is singled out for abuse whilst the rest of the family appear well cared for. The most common forms of deliberate injury are shown in Fig. 53; they are:

1   Bruising, especially of the face and trunk which are rare sites for accidental injury. Bruises may be multiple and of different ages.

2   Fractures, especially of the ribs, humerus and femur. Such fractures in infancy should always alert the doctor.

3   Head injury. Skull fracture and subdural haematoma may occur together or separately. Retinal and sub-hyaloid haemor-

rhages are a common accompaniment. The most severe head injuries will causes intra-ventricular and intra-cerebral haemorrhage leading to death or permanent brain damage.

4   Burns, either from cigarettes or from holding the child close to a fire.

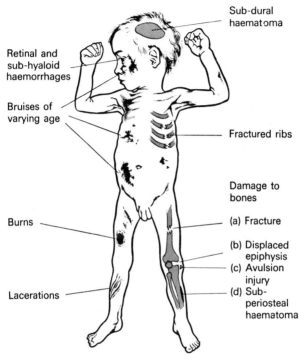

Sub-dural haematoma

Retinal and sub-hyaloid haemorrhages

Bruises of varying age

Fractured ribs

Damage to bones

Burns

(a) Fracture

(b) Displaced epiphysis

(c) Avulsion injury

Lacerations

(d) Sub-periosteal haematoma

Fig. 53. Injuries sustained by battered babies.

The doctor's suspicions should be aroused by the history if (a) there has been an inexplicable delay in seeking medical advice, which may even be as long as a few days; (b) the explanation given for the injuries is not compatible with their severity. For example, a baby's skull does not fracture if he rolls off the sofa on to a carpeted floor. If there is any reasonable suspicion of deliberate injury the child must be admitted to hospital for his own safety. A careful clinical record of bruises and other skin lesions must be made, with drawings and photographs. A skeletal X-ray survey may show unsuspected fractures at various stages of healing.

The doctor's function is not to act as detective or judge, even less as public prosecutor, but to safeguard his patient and help the family. The NSPCC and social services department may well be enlisted to help, and in some areas the police adopt a constructive attitude. Court action may be necessary to take a child into the care of the local authority if the risk of further assault is felt to be substantial. Further abuse occurs in up to 20% of cases, but the recurrence rate is a sensitive index of the effectiveness of management. If there is skilled, intensive, continuous help for these families, recurrence can be altogether avoided.

COT DEATH (sudden unexplained death of infancy)

The sudden death of an infant which is unexpected by history, and in which a thorough post mortem examination fails to demonstrate an adequate cause, occurs in just under 3 per 1000 live births. In the United Kingdom cot deaths constitute about one fifth of infant deaths.

Most occur at home between the ages of 4 weeks and 4 months, in urban rather than rural areas, during the night, and in late winter and early spring, when community respiratory infections are most prevalent. They are frequently preceded by symptoms of minor illness, they are more common in males, in twins, in infants of low birth weight, and in the socially and economically deprived. The infants' mothers tend to be younger and to have had more children when compared to controls. They do not keep antenatal clinic appointments for themselves or follow up clinic appointments for the babies.

Substantial proof is lacking for the many hypotheses which have been proposed to explain cot deaths.

Further reading

Apley J. & MacKeith R.C. (1968) Accidents to children. Chapter 7, *The Child and his Symptoms*. Blackwell Scientific Publications, Oxford.

Reid D.H.S. (1970) Treatment of the poisoned child. *Archives of Disease in Childhood*, **45,** 428.

Non-accidental injury in children. Report from B.P.A. and B.A.P.S. (1973) *British Medical Journal*, **4,** 656.

Franklin A.W. (1975) *Concerning Child Abuse*. Churchill Livingstone, Edinburgh and London.

Chapter 23

CHILDREN IN SOCIETY

The health and educational progress of a child is directly related to the home and the environment. The child of an unskilled worker (social class V) has a 50% greater chance of being born dead or with a serious physical handicap than a lawyer's child (social class I). The disadvantage is there at birth and continues throughout childhood. The social class IV or V child will have more physical illnesses, will be smaller and will read less well than the child from social class I or II. The Registrar-General's five-point grading of social class is a crude, but useful classification. Although it depends on the occupation of the father, we recognize that the father's occupation has close correlation with many other important factors including income, housing and attitudes to child rearing. In Britain the proportion of families in each social class is approximately:

I	Higher professional (usually university graduates)	5%
II	Other professional and technical	15%
III	Other non manual and skilled manual	55%
IV	Semi-skilled manual	19%
V	Unskilled manual	6%

Unsatisfactory homes are not just those where there is overt cruelty, poverty or squalor. Stress at home may result from parental discord—quarrelling and separations, one parent families, and children who have been put in the care of the wrong parent after divorce. It may result from parental illness—a dying or chronically handicapped mother, a mentally ill father—or just from parental inadequacy—work-shy parents, drunken parents and those who have given up the struggle of trying to be satisfactory parents.

The doctor sees the childhood casualties of these situations: poor development, illness and behaviour problems, or children who have to stay in hospital because of the home situation rather than the severity of the illness. The teacher sees the casualties also; unhappy children, delinquent children and children with school problems.

Elaborate local authority medical and social services exist particularly for such children. But all too often the services are best used by the child of well-informed middle-class parents, while the socially disadvantaged child cannot use them, because his parents either do not know or do not care. Therefore all medical and para-medical staff have a constant duty to detect children in need or in distress and to see that they have the opportunity to benefit from the help that is available.

Some of the more important of these services are summarized in this chapter. As a result of the 1974 reorganization some of the services described are undergoing major changes, and other new services are developing.

COMMUNITY MEDICAL SERVICES

Health Visitors

These are registered nurses who also hold a midwifery qualification and a health visitor's certificate. They are employed by the Area Health Authority though an increasing number are being allocated to group general practices and a few have hospital attachments. They are responsible for family health, and particularly that of mothers and children. Their job is to prevent illness and handicap by the early detection of problems and mobilization of services to deal with those problems. Their duties range from screening 9-month-old infants for deafness and advising mothers of young children, to being the friend and helper of old folk who live alone.

Child Health Centres (Infant Welfare Clinics)

These are organized by the Area Health Authority and are staffed by health visitors and ancillary workers. Most of the doctors who work at these centres do so on a part time sessional basis and may be general practitioners. Their role is a supervisory one; they aim to provide routine medical examination of infants and pre-school children and to ensure optimal physical, emotional and mental development for the child. They provide immunization services and health education for new mothers, as well as advising and supporting those who have problems. 90% of babies attend such a centre at least once in the first year; but after the age of 2 attendance drops sharply.

EDUCATION AND THE SCHOOL HEALTH SERVICE

The principal school medical officer in any area is the Area Medical Officer. However, the school health services are separated off to some extent from the rest of his responsibilities so that those in the service can work in close collaboration with the education department and local paediatricians.

School medical officers, many of whom are part-time workers, are responsible for identifying schoolchildren with disorders which are likely to interfere with their development, education and happiness. The traditional annual 5-minute inspection of every child is being replaced by more detailed assessment of a few selected children about whom the school teachers are worried.

The school health service provides a large number of 'School Clinics' held in education premises which supplement and sometimes duplicate hospital outpatient clinics. Many towns provide regular schoolchild ophthalmology, ENT, orthopaedic and dental clinics as well as physiotherapy, orthoptic, and speech therapy facilities. It is probable that these clinics will become more closely linked with general hospitals in the future.

The education department has to provide *Special School* facilities for 11 groups of children who require special education. These are for children who are:
Deaf,
Partially hearing,
Blind,
Partially sighted,

Epileptic,
ESN (N)—educationally subnormal (normal),
ESN (S)—educationally subnormal (severe),
Maladjusted (psychological disorders),
Speech problems (other than the deaf),
Physically handicapped (e.g. cerebral palsy or spina bifida),
Delicate (a small and decreasing number of children who do not fit into the other categories but cannot manage at normal school, e.g. because of intractable asthma).

Most areas will have adequate facilities for children who are ESN or physically handicapped—the disorders are common. But for less common disorders the child may have to be a boarder far from home and the local authority pays. For instance, there are at present only 2 schools of 'grammar school' level for blind children in England.

The special schools play an important role in the welfare of handicapped children; but most parents want their child to attend a normal school if at all possible. The extra staff and facilities of the special school are outweighed in their minds by the inconvenience, the social stigma of being different, and the lower academic standard of most special schools.

Nursery Schools

These exist as separate schools or as nursery classes attached to primary schools. They cater for children aged 3 to 5 and are run by specially trained teachers assisted by nursery assistants and nurses. They aim to encourage a child's development and learning by play, stimulation and physical activity.

There is a great shortage of these schools and classes, and at present under 5% of children can be accommodated; the number who would benefit is many times that proportion. Priority is given to children with social or medical handicap, and to those with mothers who go out to work.

DEPARTMENT OF SOCIAL SERVICES

The Social Services Department is responsible for the care and/or supervision of children up to 18 years in a variety of circumstances.

A child may be accommodated by the local authority if he cannot be cared for by his parents or guardians temporarily or permanently, by reason of their illness or death, or because the child has been abandoned or lost. In certain circumstances, the local authority may be designated a 'fit person' to assume parental rights in order to provide security and protection for the child. Parental rights may be given to the local authority by the Court (usually the Juvenile Court) in which case, a child is said to be the subject of a *Care Order*. In Britain over 90,000 children are in care. Grounds for a care order include health impairment, neglect of proper development, ill treatment, moral danger, failure to attend school, incitement to crime, or being beyond the control of parent or guardian. The child has to be in need of care and control which is unlikely to be received unless a care order is made. The local authority tries to keep or place children with their own parents, relatives or friends whether care is temporary permanent, voluntary or through a court order. When this is not possible local authority accommodation is used; it includes:

1 *Foster Homes*: Ordinary family homes which can welcome an extra child or two, whether for a succession of short stays or as a long term addition to the household.

2 *Children's Homes*: usually run on 'family' lines, aiming to provide as normal an upbringing as possible despite frequent changes of staff. They contain a higher proportion of difficult or handicapped children than foster homes. Ninety-five per cent of children in these homes still have a living parent, so that many are visited regularly or may be reunited with their parents for weekends or longer periods in the future.

3 *Hostels for Working Children*

4 *Residential Nurseries*

5 *Community Homes* (formerly approved schools): Children may now be placed directly into these homes.

6 *Mentally Handicapped Children*: Local authorities have a general responsibility for providing accommodation; this may be in the form of a special home or hostel.

Children are also supervised in their own homes either on a voluntary basis or as a result of a court *Supervision Order*: the social worker's prime aim here is to prevent family break-up and to try to help with problems of care, physical and emotional. The social worker is always glad to work as part of a team with others involved with the family, e.g. health visitors, do. teachers.

The social services department is also responsible for supervising children placed privately with foster parents. People who look after other people's children, whether on a day (child day care, childminder) or residential (foster) basis, must register with their local social services department, even though they may be paid direct by the parent.

Day Nurseries

These are for pre-school children and cater for 2 main groups of children (1) those who require daytime care whilst their parents are at work or ill—particularly those who only have a single parent. (2) Children from poor quality homes where stimulation and company are lacking. The number of day nurseries is few and the demand large. This has led to groups of parents forming their own centres for pre-school children, variously named *Play groups*, play centres, crèches, etc. Most of these groups require considerable parent participation and organization and at present are mainly run by middle-class parents for their middle-class children.

VOLUNTARY SERVICES

The statutory services are supplemented by a large number of voluntary and charitable organizations. Some of these organizations were amongst the first to provide any help for disadvantaged children. The NSPCC (National Society for the Prevention of Cruelty to Children) continues its historic role of providing support and advice for families under stress. Barnardo's continues to provide good happy residential care for homeless and handicapped children. Other organizations are relatively new. The Spastics Society provides medical and educational services for children with cerebral palsy in addition to sponsoring a large research programme.

ADOPTION

Couples wishing to adopt a baby should approach either their local authority or a registered adoption society. Each agency tends to have its own requirements, for instance attachment to a particular religious denomination or an age limit—it is difficult to adopt a child if you are over 40. The agencies' main concern will be relationships within the family, but it is also important for applicants to have a steady income, a settled home and satisfactory health. Once accepted the applicants have to wait anything from a few months to three years, until a suitable baby is placed with them. A child of any age up to 17 may be adopted but the most usual placements are of illegitimate babies. The natural mother, and in some circumstances the father, is asked to sign a form agreeing to the adoption. There is a minimum three months probationary period, during which the natural mother can claim the baby back; about 2% do. During this period the applicants will be visited by a social worker as will all the people concerned in the adoption. At the end of this time, if parental consents are signed and confirmed and reports on the adoptive home are satisfactory, the Adoption Order will be made in Court. The child is now a full member of the adoptive family; he takes their name and has all the rights of a natural child (except that he cannot inherit a title!).

Medical examinations are required for both parents, for the baby before placement and again before the adoption hearing. It is essential to explain and discuss any suspected handicaps with the prospective parents. Parents are also advised to inform their child from the beginning that they are adopted and to explain this regularly and more fully as the child's understanding increases.

The increased tolerance shown by society to unmarried mothers, and the increased financial and practical support available for them have resulted in fewer babies being offered for adoption. There is now a shortage of healthy non-coloured babies for adoption, and an excess of childless couples wishing to adopt.

Pregnant women seeking advice about adoption should be advised to approach their social services department or a recognized voluntary organization specializing in helping the unmarried mother.

A leaflet for prospective adopters which gives the necessary details about adoption societies is available from the Association of British Adoption Agencies, 4 Southampton Row, London WC1 B 4AA.

LAWS RELATING TO THE YOUNG

For legal purposes a child remains a 'child' up to the age of 14, is a 'young person' up to 17, and is an adult over 18. However many laws become operative at other ages.

School

School education is compulsory for children over the age of 5. Children may not leave until they are 16.

Work

Children may not be employed until they are 13. Then they may be employed only between the hours of 7 am and 7 pm, and for a maximum of 2 hours on school days.

Abuse

It is an offence to:
tattoo anyone under 18,
seduce a girl under 16,
sell tobacco to a child under 16,
sell fireworks to a child under 13,
expose to fire risk (e.g. not use a fire guard) a child under 12,
give intoxicating liquor to children under 5.

Crime

Children under 10 (under 8 in Scotland) are not considered 'criminally responsible' for their misdeeds, and may be dealt with by Juvenile Courts.

The court can make (1) a 'Care Order' giving parental rights to the local authority or (2) a 'Supervision Order' which may be administered by the social services department or, if the child is over 14, by the probation department. At the age of 15 children can be sent to Borstal.

Adult courts deal with those over the age of 17. Although it is legally possible to be sent to prison for a first offence at the age of 17, it is in practice rare before the age of 20.

———

At the age of 100 the child receives a telegram of congratulation from the Queen.

Chapter 24

MORTALITY AND MORBIDITY

The pattern of illness and the causes of death in childhood are markedly different from those of adult life. Deaths and their causes have been notifiable for well over a century in Britain. Stillbirths, and more recently their causes, are also notifiable. From this information published each year by the Registrar General, it is possible to study the causes of death at different ages, the effects of such factors as sex, season, place of residence and illegitimacy and the trends in mortality over the years.

Mortality in childhood is concentrated at the beginning, and the most important statistics relate to this period. The *infant mortality rate* is the number of infants dying in the first year of life out of every 1000 born alive. *Neonatal* mortality refers to the first 4 weeks of life. The stillbirth rate is the number of babies born dead after 28 weeks gestation for every 1000 *total* births. As the causes of stillbirth have much in common with deaths in the first *week* of life, these are often combined under the term *perinatal* mortality (in 1972 this was 22 for England and Wales).

Information about non-fatal disease or handicap in childhood is less readily available, but much valuable information is provided by studies such as the Newcastle thousand families survey and the National Child Development Study.

The table and charts that follow are based on the sources mentioned, but are adapted and simplified where necessary to stress the important aspects of mortality and morbidity in childhood.

Table 16. Death rates per million in childhood, by age. England and Wales, 1972, all causes.

| | Age in years | | |
	0–1	1–4	5–14
Males	19,104	777	382
Females	14,812	709	247

It is apparent that childhood deaths are concentrated in the first year of life, and that death rates at all ages in childhood are about one third higher for boys than for girls.

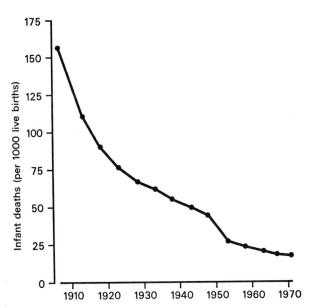

Fig. 54. *Infant Mortality* (*0–1 year*). By 1972, the infant mortality rate in England and Wales had fallen to one tenth of the level in 1900 —from 156 to 17 per 1000 live births. The present rate is amongst the lowest in the world but by no means the lowest in Europe.

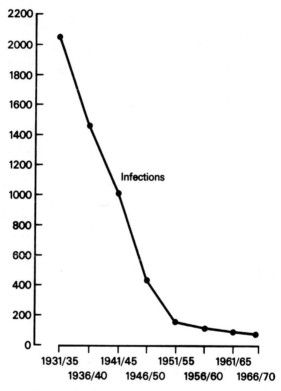

Fig. 55. *Child Mortality from Infections, 1931–1970.* There has been a dramatic decline in child deaths from infections, from over 2000 to under 100 per million children living, aged 1–14 years. The decline was as dramatic before the introduction of sulphonamides and anti-biotics as subsequently. This should be contrasted with Fig. 56.

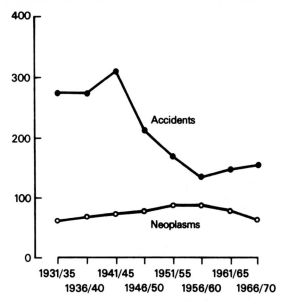

Fig. 56. *Child Mortality from Accidents and Neoplasms, 1931–1970.* Child mortality rates from accidents peaked during the 1939/45 war and subsequently declined, but are currently on the increase again. Death rates from neoplasms have not improved in the last 40 years.

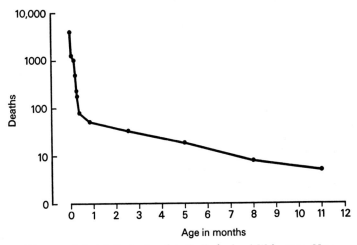

Fig. 57. *Infant deaths by day of death. England and Wales 1971.* Note that the vertical scale is logarithmic. In 1971, 4680 babies died within 24 hours of birth: 169 on the 7th day of life: only 3 or 4 on their first birthday. Efforts to reduce child mortality must be concentrated on the perinatal period.

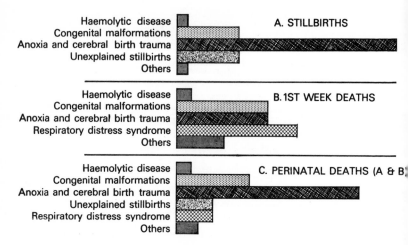

Fig. 58. *Cause of Perinatal Mortality.* More than half of all stillbirths result from difficulties at delivery. One in six is unexplained. One third of first-week deaths result from respiratory problems, mostly in pre-term babies.

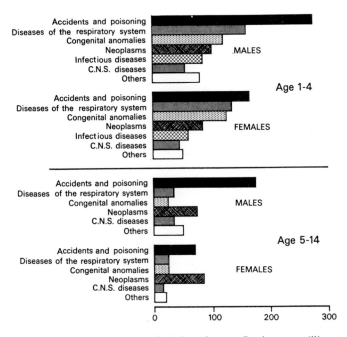

Fig. 59. *Childhood mortality after infancy, by cause. Death rate per million living, England and Wales.* Deaths are higher at ages 1–4 than at 5–14 years for all causes, and are higher in boys than in girls for almost all causes. Accidents and poisoning are the major killers in both sexes after infancy. In young children, respiratory disease and congenital anomalies come next, with neoplasms fourth. In older children, neoplasms are the second major cause of death.

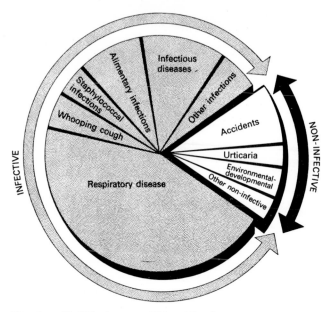

Fig. 60. *Morbidity in young children.* The data presented relate to Newcastle children in 1947–52. In the first 5 years of life, 847 children experienced 8467 episodes of ill health, an average of 2 per child each year. At other times and in other places the total amount of illness will be different, but the pattern will be similar. 80% of illnesses were infective, and two-thirds of these were respiratory.

INCIDENCE OF SOME IMPORTANT PROBLEMS

10% of 1-year-old-boys have been circumcised.

7% of 5-year-olds have had at least one convulsion.

5% of 5-year-olds have a squint.

5% of 5-year-olds have a behaviour problem.

5% of 5-year-olds have a speech or language problem.

2% of 5-year-olds have a substantial congenital defect.

16% of 7-year-olds have had tonsillectomy or adenoidectomy.

2% of 7-year-olds have had a hernia repair.

1% of 7-year-olds have had an appendicectomy.

10% of 7-year-olds wet their beds.

10% of 7-year-olds have eczema, asthma or hay fever.

13% of 7-year-olds require special schooling.

5% of 7-year-olds receive special schooling.

INCIDENCE OF SOME NOTORIOUS CONDITIONS

Many conditions about which you have learnt, and some of which you will have seen in large regional children's centres, are very rare. Professor Illingworth of Sheffield has calculated the average length of time that a British general practitioner (with a practice of 2,500 patients) would have to work to see a child presenting with one of the following conditions:

Pyloric stenosis	4	years
Mental subnormality	4	,,
Congenital heart disease	5	,,
Spina bifida	6	,,
Diabetes mellitus	6	,,
Epilepsy	6	,,
Cot death	8	,,
Intussusception	12	,,
Hydrocephalus	12	,,
Mongol	16	,,
Congenital dislocation of the hip	37	,,
Turner's syndrome	60	,,
Oesophageal atresia	75	,,

Autism	120 years
Adrenogenital syndrome	200 "
Phenylketonuria	240 "
Cretin	250 "
Malignant disease	250 "
Nephrotic syndrome	350 "
Muscular dystrophy	480 "
Haemophilia	600 "
Hirschsprung's disease	600 "
Galactosaemia	1725 "
Tay-Sachs disease	6250 "

Further reading

Davie R., Butler N.R. & Goldstein H. (1972) *From Birth to Seven*. Longman, London.

The Registrar General's Statistical review of England and Wales for the year 1972. Part I. Tables. Medical. Her Majesty's Stationery Office, London.

APPENDIXES

Appendix 1. Head circumference chart

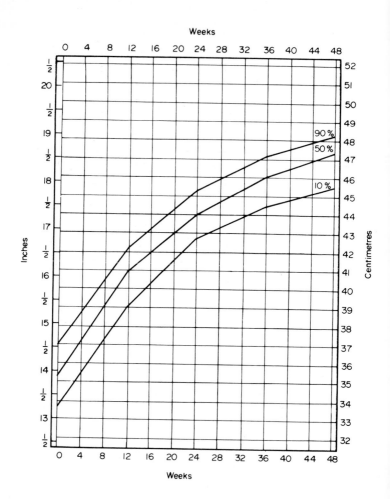

Appendix 2. Weight and height percentile table for boys

Age	Weight kg 3%	Weight kg 50%	Weight kg 97%	Height cm 3%	Height cm 50%	Height cm 97%
Birth	2.5	3.5	4.4		50	
3 months	4.4	5.7	7.2	55	60	64
6 ,,	6.2	7.8	9.8	62	66.5	71
9 ,,	7.6	9.3	11.6	66.5	71	76
12 ,,	8.4	10.3	12.8	70	75	80
15 ,,	9.0	11	13.6	73	78	84
18 ,,	9.4	11.7	14.2	75	81	87
21 ,,	9.8	12.2	14.9	78	84	90
2 years	10.2	12.7	16	80	87	93
2½ ,,	10.9	13.7	17	84	92	99
3 ,,	11.6	14.7	18	86	95	103
3½ ,,	12.5	15.8	19	90	98	106
4 ,,	13	17	20	94	101	110
4½ ,,	14	18	22	96	105	114
5 ,,	14.5	19	23	100	108	117
6 ,,	16	21	25	105	114	124
7 ,,	17	23	28	110	120	130
8 ,,	19	25	31	115	126	137
9 ,,	21	27	35	120	132	143
10 ,,	23	30	39	125	137	148
11 ,,	25	34	43	128	141	154
12 ,,	27	38	49	133	147	160
13 ,,	30	43	55	137	151	165
14 ,,	33	48	62	142	157	172
15 ,,	39	55	67	148	163	179

Head circumference (cm) for boys

	3%	50%	97%
Birth	33	35	38
12 months	45	47	49
18 months	46	49	51
2 years	47	50	52
3 ,,	48	50	53
5 ,,	49	51	54
8 ,,	50	52	55
12 ,,	51	54	56
14 ,,	53	56	58

Appendix 3. Weight and height percentile table for girls

Age	Weight kg			Height cm		
	3%	50%	97%	3%	50%	97%
Birth	2.5	3.5	4.4		50	
3 months	4.4	5.6	7.2	55	60	65
6 ,,	6.2	7.8	9.8	62	67	72
9 ,,	7.8	9.2	11.6	65	71	76
12 ,,	8.4	10.3	12.8	70	75	80
15 ,,	9.0	11.0	13.6	73	78	84
18 ,,	9.4	11.6	14.2	75	81	87
21 ,,	9.8	12.2	14.8	78	84	90
2 years	10.2	12.7	15.5	80	87	93
2½ ,,	11	13.7	16.7	84	92	99
3 ,,	11.6	14.7	18	85	95	104
3½ ,,	12	15	19	90	97	105
4 ,,	13	16	20	93	100	108
4½ ,,	14	17	21	96	104	112
5 ,,	15	18	22	99	107	116
6 ,,	16	19	25	104	114	123
7 ,,	18	22	28	109	120	129
8 ,,	19	24	32	114	125	135
9 ,,	21	26	36	118	130	142
10 ,,	23	29	41	123	135	148
11 ,,	25	33	46	128	141	156
12 ,,	28	37	52	133	147	161
13 ,,	31	41	57	139	153	167
14 ,,	36	46	62	145	158	170
15 ,,	40	51	67	149	160	172

Head circumference (cm) for girls

	3%	50%	97%
Birth	33	35	38
12 months	43	46	48
18 months	45	47	50
2 years	46	48	51
3 ,,	47	49	52
5 ,,	48	50	53
8 ,,	50	52	54
12 ,,	51	53	56
14 ,,	52	54	57

Appendix 4. Teeth

There are 20 deciduous teeth and 32 permanent teeth

Deciduous		Appearance
Central Incisor	lower	6–10 months
	upper	7–10 ,,
Lateral Incisor	upper	8–10 ,,
	lower	12–18 ,,
First Molar		12–18 ,,
Canine		16–20 ,,
Second Molar		20–30 ,,

Permanent teeth appear from the 6th year. The first molars and central incisors appear first. All teeth have appeared by the age of 14 except the third molars. Teeth appear a few months earlier in girls.

A fluoride content of 1 part per million in the water results in 30–50% less caries. Therefore, in the many areas in which fluoride content is low, a fluoride supplement is advisable, particularly during the first 8 years of life.

Appendix 5. Chronological order of appearance of osseous centres

	Birth	6 months	1 yr	2	3	4	5

Shoulder	Head of humerus (3 months)		Greater tuberosity				
Elbow			Capitulum				Head of radius
Hand		Hamate (4 months) Capitate (6 months)	Ep. radius		Triquetral Ep. meta- carpals Ep. phal- anges	Lunate	Trapezium Scapho' 1
Hip		Head of femur (9 months)				Greater trochanter	
Knee Ep. femur & tibia						Head of fibula	Patella
Foot Cuboid		Lat. cunei- form Ep. tibia	Ep. fibula	Intermedi- ate cunei- form Ep. metatarsals	Med. cunei- form Navicular		

The new centres of ossification which appear at each year are shown in black.

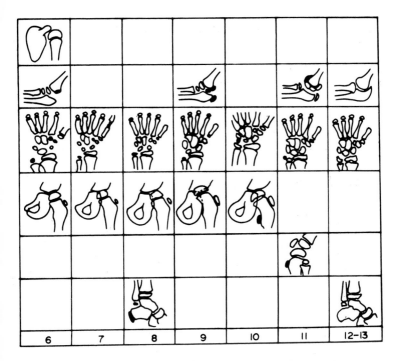

6	7	8	9	10	11	12-13

Union head
and tuber-
osity

Int. epi-condyle			Trochlea Oleranon		Ext. epicon-dyle

Trapezoid Ep. ulna				Pisiform	Styloid ulna

	Union is-chium and pubis			Ep. lesser trochanter	

					Tibial tu-bercle

		Ep. os calcis			

Appendix 6. Developmental milestones*

Posture and movement

3 months

Prone: rests on forearms, lifts up head and chest.

Pulled to sit: head bobs forward, then held erect.

Held standing: sags at knees.

6 months

Prone: lifts self up on extended arms.

Pulls self to sit, and sits erect with support.

Held standing: takes weight on legs.

9 months

Prone: wriggles or crawls.

Sits unsupported for 10 minutes.

Held standing: bounces or stamps.

1 year

Crawls on all fours.

Walks round furniture stepping sideways. Walks with hands held.

Stands alone for a second or two.

1½ years

Walks alone and can pick up a toy from floor without falling.

2 years

Runs.

Walks up and down stairs two feet to a step.

3 years

Walks upstairs one foot per step, and down two feet per step.

Stands on one foot momentarily

4 years

Walks up and down stairs one foot per step.

Stands on one foot for 5 seconds.

5 years

Skips. Hops.

Stands on one foot with arms folded for 5 seconds.

Vision and manipulation

Vision: alert, watches movement of adult.

Follows dangling toy held 6 inches from face.

Hands: loosely open.

Watches rolling ball 2 yards away.

Reaches out for toys and takes in palmar grasp, puts to mouth.

Looks for toys that are dropped.

Scissor grasp and transfer to other hand before placing object in mouth.

Drops toys deliberately and watches where they go.

Index finger approach to tiny objects, then pincer grasp.

Builds tower of three cubes.
Scribbles.

Builds tower of six cubes.

Builds tower of nine cubes.
Copies a ○.

Builds three steps from six cubes (after demonstration).
Copies a ○ and ×.

Draws a man.
Copies ○, × and □.

* Average age of achievements

276

Hearing and speech	*Social behaviour*
Quietens to interesting sounds. Chuckles and coos when pleased.	Shows pleasure appropriately.
Localizes soft sounds 18 inches lateral to either ear. Makes double syllable sounds and tuneful noises.	Alert, interested. Still friendly with strangers.
Brisk localization of soft sounds 3 foot lateral to either ear. Babbles tunefully.	Distinguishes strangers and shows apprehension. Chews solids.
Understands simple commands. Babbles incessantly.	Cooperates with dressing, e.g. holding up arms. Waves bye bye.
Uses several words, sound labels.	Drinks from cup using two hands. Demands constant mothering.
Joins words together in simple phrases, as sound ideas.	Uses spoon. Indicates toilet needs, dry by day.
Speaks in sentences. Gives full name.	Eats with spoon and fork. Can undress with assistance. Dry by night.
Talks a lot. Speech contains many infantile substitutions.	Dresses and undresses with assistance.
Fluent speech with few infantile substitutions.	Dresses and undresses alone. Washes and dries face and hands.

INDEX